The Anesthesiologist's Guide to the OR: *Prepped*

The Anesthesiologist's Guide to the OR: *Prepped*

Richard P. Dutton, M.D.
Assistant Professor and Staff Anesthesiologist
National Naval Medical Center
Bethesda, Maryland

Adam D. Goldstein, M.D.
Resident in Anesthesiology
National Naval Medical Center
Bethesda, Maryland

With
Robert M. Gantt, M.D.
Paul F. Lennon, M.D.
Paul A. Pudimat, M.D.

Little, Brown and Company
Boston   New York   Toronto   London

Copyright © 1995 by Richard P. Dutton and Adam D. Goldstein

First Edition
Second Printing

Library of Congress Cataloging-in-Publication Data

Dutton, Richard P.
    The anesthesiologist's guide to the OR : prepped / Richard P.
Dutton, Adam D. Goldstein, with Robert M. Gantt, Paul F. Lennon,
Paul A. Pudimat.
       p.   cm.
    Includes bibliographical references and index.
    ISBN 0-316-19958-3
    1. Anesthesiology--Handbooks, manuals, etc. 2. Surgery,
Operative--Handbooks, manuals, etc. I. Goldstein, Adam D.
II. Title.
    [DNLM: 1. Anesthesia--methods--handbook. 2. Surgery, Operative-
-handbooks. 3. Anesthesiology--handbooks. WO 231 D981a 1994]
RD82.2.D88 1994
617.9'6--dc20
DNLM/DLC
for Library of Congress   94-27187
                                                    CIP

Printed in the United States of America

RRD-VA

Editorial: Nancy Megley
Copyeditor: Jean Webb Bonnyman
Indexer: Elizabeth Willingham
Designer: Cate Rickard
Composition and Production: Silverchair Science + Communications

To our beautiful, fantastic, beloved wives,
Greykell and Amy,
who make our whole lives great

Contents

Preface

Ever wonder what position a percutaneous nephrostomy tube placement is done in? How long a laparoscopic Nissen fundoplication is going to take? How much blood the patient will lose during a total knee replacement?

We've had these questions, too, especially the first time we saw our names next to such cases on the daily surgical schedule. In fact, we've had many questions about the surgical procedures we haven't done before— usually *basic* questions. And where can we turn for answers?

As residents, we could ask our staff anesthesiologist. This would yield a generally useful answer, although sometimes short on practical detail if he or she was a long time out of training. Admitting ignorance was painful, but at least it kept us from being an attraction at M & M conference.

Occasionally we were able to debrief a senior resident first and get the nuts and bolts ahead of time. Finding a colleague who had done the case before was sometimes a challenge, and this approach could backfire when the resident pretended to know more than he or she did.

We also tried asking the surgeons, and the OR nurses, and the scrub technicians. They had many useful comments about the cases but very little perspective on what we, the anesthesiologists, really needed to know.

Finally, there was the literature. Textbooks and journal articles are great for understanding physiology, demographics, and pharmacodynamics but are often very poor for the fundamental management of a given case. Even when they do address things like patient positioning, the information is often so buried in other minutiae that it is impossible to extract. And it's hard to put a copy of Miller in your back pocket.

Hence, this book. *Prepped* is intended to be a practical, portable reference for the things you need to know about any given procedure. It is written for the junior resident or student nurse anesthetist making the first round of the surgical services and focuses on what you really need to know: positioning, estimated blood loss, surgical time, suitability for regional techniques, and indicated monitoring. It discusses each case individually and lists the complications you are likely to encounter. The cases are organized by surgical service for easy access.

Before we begin with the technical information, we would also like to share Dutton's Three Rules of Anesthesia:

1. Understand the surgical procedure.
2. Titrate to effect.
3. Never refuse a lunch break.

Why is it so important to understand the surgical procedure? First, the surgeons are the only reason for your existence. Very few patients come to the hospital just for an anesthetic. We may feel personal repugnance at catering to the every whim of some pajama-clad prima donna, but let's face it: We're a service industry. Knowing the surgical procedure will help you make it go faster. The anesthesia will be appropriate, the table will be the right height, and the patient will wake up when you want him or her to. Sudden blood loss will not catch you unaware, nor will demands for obscure drugs, bizarre positions, or unusual monitoring. As the surgeon comes to realize that you are also concerned with the case as a whole and not just the stock ticker buried among your electronics, he or she will develop a higher opinion of you, and your professional relationship will improve. In academia this will mean less friction and more research time. In private practice this will mean more money.

Patient care will also improve. There will be less waiting around, and you will be more confident and knowledgeable. You will be able to answer questions for the patient and family and give them a good idea preoperatively about the likely hospital course. Morbidity will decline, because you will be giving the appropriate anesthetic with the appropriate monitoring and the appropriate vigilance to the case's likely trouble spots. All in all, the more you know about the surgical procedure, the better.

The best way to find out about a given procedure is to do a few. Direct experience leads to learning, after all, and the need to learn about a wide variety of anesthetics is the reason your residency is 3 years long. This kind of on-the-job training has its drawbacks, however, which are readily apparent the first time the vascular surgeon cross-clamps your patient's aorta when you're not looking.

Prepped is the second best way to learn about cases—one that will help you avoid the major morbidities associated with the experiential method. The information in *Prepped* may even help you impress the surgeons, dazzle your staff anesthesiologist, and find lifelong happiness and fulfillment. Or so we hope.

R.P.D.
A.D.G.

Acknowledgments

We credit the following people for their invaluable assistance, without which you would probably be reading some lesser tome, albeit written by more famous people:

Liz Thompson, formerly of Little, Brown and Company, for the "power lunch" that got the ball rolling.

Nancy Megley, also of Little, Brown and Company, for picking up the ball and running with it.

Dan Beisel, of Medical Art Design, for illustrating the ball. (OK, that's enough of that metaphor.) Dan actually provided the illustrations for this book, and in an amazingly short time, too.

Our collaborators at the National Naval Medical Center: Drs. Gantt, Lennon, and Pudimat. These amazing talents are each credited specifically in the chapters they worked on, but we thank them here as well for all their time and effort spent reviewing the book as a whole.

And while we're at it: the rest of the Department of Anesthesia at the National Naval Medical Center. You know who you are. We appreciate your patience with us while this book was assembling itself, and we admire the self-restraint you displayed when we were looting your offices for reference material. Thanks!

About This Book

Prepped is organized in as user-friendly a fashion as we could contrive. The procedures are divided by service and organized within each section from common cases to more obscure ones. We have not listed every conceivable variation of every conceivable case but instead have tried to focus on the most common and most typical procedures of each surgical specialty.

Which brings us to an important caveat: Nothing is ever the same. Surgeons vary, institutions vary, anesthesiologists vary, and patients vary. Strange things sometimes happen. At one hospital we know of, a vasovasostomy (reversal of a vasectomy) is a 6-hour case involving a microscope and a general anesthetic. At another hospital it is a 1-hour case usually done under spinal anesthesia. Obviously, it is hard to incorporate both of these extremes in a brief discussion. We have tried throughout to take a middle-of-the-road approach applicable to most procedures in most teaching institutions. If you discover we are wrong about something, don't panic! Make a note of it in the book, and move on. You'll be ready for it next time.

The first chapter is called Generic Stuff, and that's exactly what it's full of: short descriptions of many of the simple, yet important, aspects of your job—things that apply to many cases. We refer back to these pages throughout the rest of the book, so you'll probably become quite familiar with them.

The other chapters discuss the common procedures performed on a specific surgical service and begin with a discussion of the fundamental features of that service—information that will be applicable to most, if not all, of the specific procedures discussed.

The discussions of specific procedures begin with a short description of what the surgeons will be doing, as you might see it from the head of the table. This is followed by comments in seven categories common to all procedures: patient position, estimated time, estimated blood loss, need for muscle relaxation, appropriate monitoring, likely postoperative analgesic requirements, and anesthetic techniques.

Patient position is an obvious thing to know about any procedure and one of the most important for the anesthesiologist. Where to put the IV, where to put the BP cuff, which side of the mouth to tape the endotracheal tube on, and so forth will all depend on the patient's position during the surgery. Even knowing where on the body to put the ECG pads can save you time (and ECG pads!) later. We have also included a few pages in Chapter 1 describing the common positions, along with illustrations. A picture, after all, is worth a thousand words.

Estimated time is one of the most variable of the data points. Time is highly dependent on the surgeon and the institution, and our estimates may be off by hours in some cases. In general, though, if a hernia repair at your institution takes longer than we say it should, then it's a safe bet that a cholecystectomy by the same surgeon will be off by a similar factor. With a few cases under your belt and a little bit of careful observation, you'll be able to use our predictions with some accuracy.

Estimated blood loss also varies from surgeon to surgeon and patient to patient. We have tried to give a rough idea of what to expect so you can plan your preoperative assessment, monitoring, anesthetic technique, and postoperative care accordingly. Again, once you learn about a particular surgeon, you'll be able to accurately predict the blood loss in future cases. Chapter 1 discusses considerations for cases in which a large blood loss is expected.

The need for muscle relaxation is a surgical consideration that affects your anesthetic plan as much as any other factor. Some cases require muscle relaxation for exposure, some cases require it because of the delicacy of the surgery, and in some cases it must be specifically avoided! We help you decide which is which.

Appropriate monitoring is something you often have to decide early in the morning, when experienced advice may be hard to find. Obviously, the patient's degree of illness will have a great deal to do with your thought process on this subject, but we can at least tell you whether you should be deciding between adding a Foley catheter or a transesophageal echo. Again, common monitoring choices are summarized in Chapter 1.

Postoperative pain management is one of the great recent advances in anesthesia practice. Good analgesia begins intraoperatively: If you know what the patient is likely to be experiencing when he or she wakes up, you will be able to give the best possible anesthetic. The various options are described in Chapter 1.

This book is particularly helpful about anesthetic techniques. We simply describe the more obvious anesthetic choices for each procedure so that you can counsel the patient appropriately. And your staff will be impressed by your flexibility.

Finally, and most important, we provide a brief commentary on the likely trouble spots of the case. It might not have occurred to you to read up on hyponatremia before anesthetizing that TURP patient, but it will if you scout the case out here first. Good luck!

The Anesthesiologist's Guide to the OR: *Prepped*

Generic Stuff

POSITIONING: THE OPERATING ROOM TABLE

Figuring out in advance what position the surgeon is going to want the patient in, and how to get the patient there, is an easy way to make yourself look good. Usually this position is achieved after the block or endotracheal tube is in, with the patient anesthetized and basically unable to help. Occasionally, though, the patient is allowed to position himself first and then be anesthetized (e.g., monitored anesthesia care [MAC] cases, prone spinals, or the rare laminectomy).

Before putting a patient on the OR table, though, it is important to understand how the cursed thing works. Figure 1-1 shows a generic OR table that you will surely recognize. It may be powered by hand cranking or by electricity, but the basic maneuvers will be the same. You should play around with an empty table some time, just for yucks, until you have figured out all of the common manipulations.

The pedal on the left side, as you face the bed from the patient's head, is for locking and unlocking the bed. When it is up, the bed will roll across the floor with all the grace and maneuverability of, say, a large refrigerator. When the pedal is down the bed will not move at all and should be rock steady. If it's not, it's because you've put the brakes down while parked on top of something—typically a power cord—and you should correct the situation before starting any surgery. Nothing aggravates the "Captain of the Operating Room" more than having the field jiggle every time someone leans on the bed. Learn to check that the bed is locked after any change in position.

The pedal on the right side controls the height of the table. Pump on it to make the table go up; press it all the way down to make the table go down. Make sure the bed is locked first.

The crank on the left side is for Trendelenburg or reverse Trendelenburg. It tips the entire platform either head-down or foot-down and is commonly used to provide the surgeon a level field, to move abdominal viscera clos-

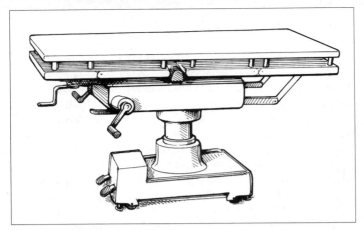

Fig. 1-1. Generic operating room table.

er or further away, or to provide more blood to the heart when the pressure is low. (Trendelenburg is your friend!)

The crank next to the Trendelenburg crank—the one facing you at the head of the bed—is for the kidney rest. Winding it up produces a bump in the middle of the table. This feature has limited applicability, but it is good to know where it is when you're actually doing a kidney operation.

The crank on the right side of the bed controls a variety of features, selected by the lever that faces you. *Back Up* bends the table in the middle, leaving the lower portion level and raising the upper portion, all the way to 90 degrees if that's what you want. *Flex* bends the table at the same joint but both parts at once; in one direction both the feet and the head get lower, while the middle gets higher; in the opposite direction the feet and head rise while the middle sinks. *Foot Down* does just that—lowers the footpiece from level all the way to −110 degrees. *Tilt* turns the bed either right or left side down and is usually used off and on during a case to provide the surgeon with the best possible view of the patient's innards.

POSITIONING: THE PATIENT

The following are the common surgical positions, expressed as both pictures and words. The **boldface**

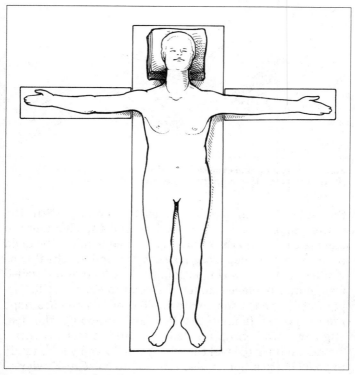

Fig. 1-2. Supine position.

words are the ones used in the rest of the text to refer to that position.

Supine position (Fig. 1-2) is far and away the most common. Patients lie flat on their backs on the operating table, arms extended to the sides on the armboards, and head elevated into "sniffing" position on a pillow. The arms should not be abducted more than 90 degrees away from the body and must rest easily on the armboards. Pressure points to watch for are under the elbows and under the buttocks. Extra padding on the bed is recommended for any case longer than about 2 hours.

Supine, arms tucked, head back, neck extended, shoulders raised, semi-sitting position (Fig. 1-3) is the classic one for thyroid surgery, many ear, nose, and throat (ENT) operations, and—with the head turned to

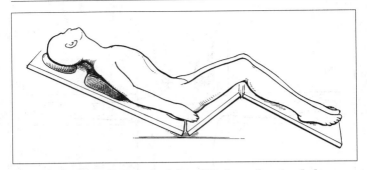

Fig. 1-3. Supine, arms tucked, head back, neck extended, shoulders raised, semi-sitting "beach chair" position.

the side—carotid endarterectomy. Starting with the patient supine, a roll is placed behind the shoulders to elevate them, and the pillow is removed to allow the head to drop back. (Keep close track of the endotracheal tube while this maneuvering is going on!) A "doughnut" rolled from gauze is placed under the head to keep it still. The patient is then made comfortable (and venous drainage improved) by flexing the bed and dropping the foot slightly, producing an "easy chair" effect. A little Trendelenburg to level the surgical field and you're ready to go. (This position is also referred to as semi-Fowler's.) The arms are tucked at the sides so the surgeons can stand on either side of the bed. Make sure all your IVs and monitors are still working *before* the surgical prep begins. Once the drapes go up, getting to either arm is going to be a pain. Consider using a "toboggan" to protect the arms from the surgeon; this is a piece of metal shaped, oddly enough, like a toboggan that tucks under the mattress and curves up over the arm, holding it at the patient's side.

Lithotomy position (Fig. 1-4) is used for any operation on the perineum, including prostatectomies, hemorrhoid resections, and vaginal hysterectomies. Beginning with the patient in supine position, the legs are elevated and separated and the feet placed in stirrups on either side of the bed. Trendelenburg is often added to tip the surgical field up a little and provide a better view for the surgeons. Pressure points to watch for are around the ankles—where the stirrups fit—and on the lateral side of

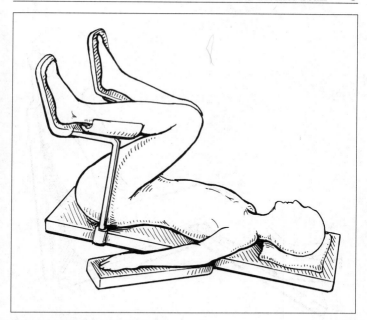

Fig. 1-4. Lithotomy position.

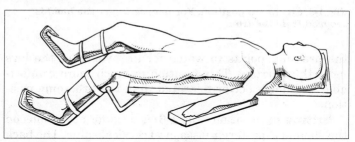

Fig. 1-5. Low stirrups. Also known as Allen stirrups.

the knees, where the stirrup pole can connect with the common peroneal nerve. The *extreme* lithotomy position, with the knees folded up toward the chest, makes it difficult for the patient to breathe spontaneously. General anesthesia, with an endotracheal tube, is a must.

Low stirrups (Fig. 1-5) are used to get the legs out of the way so that a surgeon can stand at the foot of the bed during certain abdominal operations. The legs are separated and the feet placed in stirrups that are at or below the height of the table. As with the lithotomy position,

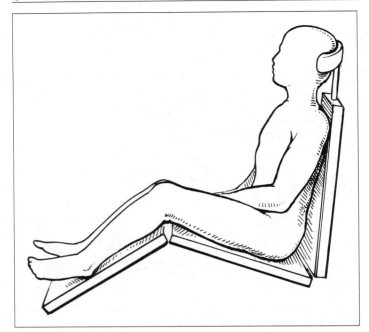

Fig. 1-6. Sitting up position. For neurosurgery the head is secured from the front.

the pressure points to watch for are wherever the legs meet the stirrups. This position is much more comfortable and much better tolerated than the lithotomy position.

Sitting up position (Fig. 1-6) is used for operations on the shoulder, posterior fossa, and cervical spine. The back of the bed is put all the way up to near 90 degrees, a little negative flex is added to raise the knees, and the foot is dropped slightly. The patient is either moved to the operative side of the bed, allowing the shoulder to hang off, or the headpiece is removed and the patient's head supported on a lower profile "horseshoe" that fits into the same slots. In either case the object is to leave the shoulder hanging free in space with the rest of the body somehow supported. Posterior fossa craniotomies are done in a similar position but with the head flexed sharply forward and secured with Mayfield tongs. The arms are tucked at the sides or secured across the patient's abdomen (take

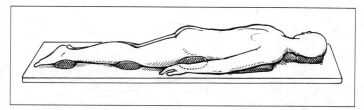

Fig. 1-7. Prone position. The bed may also be flexed to achieve the "jackknife" position, or the foot lowered to allow you to move the patient down to a kneeling position.

care that the elbows don't rest on the side rails of the bed). As always, you will want to keep a close eye on your endotracheal tube during the positioning process to make sure it stays unkinked. The same applies to any IVs that you're particularly fond of or expect to use later in the case. Think about the potential for venous air embolization whenever the surgical field is higher than the right atrium, as it is in this position.

Prone position (Fig. 1-7) is used for laminectomies, scoliosis surgery, and the like. The patient is anesthetized on the stretcher, the endotracheal tube is carefully secured, and then the patient is flipped onto the adjoining OR table. The head is usually turned to the side, with the ear resting in a gauze doughnut. The rib cage rests on two long, firm rolls, allowing the abdomen to hang free. The hips rest on the well-padded table. Padding is placed beneath the kneecaps and under the ankles. The bed is sometimes flexed slightly and then the foot raised to put comfortable bends in the hips and knees. The arms may be tucked at the sides (watch your lines and monitors!) or brought forward on armboards (pad under the elbows!). In the latter case, make sure that the shoulder is extended no more than 90 degrees. In male patients you will also want to check the location of the scrotum and penis before beginning the prep; Mr. Happy can become Mr. Unhappy very quickly if pinched between the patient and the bed. In female patients you should make sure that the breasts are not compressed. A variety of special frames and devices exist for facilitating the positioning of back surgery patients; if you see a device you haven't seen before in the OR, it would be wise to familiarize yourself with it before bringing the

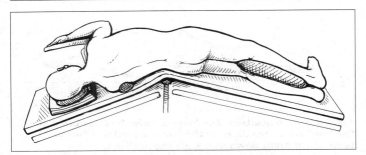

Fig. 1-8. Lateral position. If the bed is flat, rather than flexed, this is the "park bench" position.

patient in. When turning an anesthetized patient over, you will probably want to keep your anesthetic light (but the patient paralyzed) until after you see what happens to the blood pressure.

Lateral position (Fig. 1-8) is used for everything from craniotomies to hip surgery, with modifications added depending on the organ of interest. Basically, the patient is anesthetized and then turned on the side. The head will be in tongs for a neurologic case, with the headpiece of the bed removed. In other cases the head will rest on a stack of sheets, with a doughnut under the ear; the object here is to elevate the head enough to keep the neck straight with the spine. The patient lies on his or her side, with both arms extended to the front. An axillary roll—often made by wrapping a towel around a liter bag of IV fluid—is placed under the patient just south of the axilla to keep pressure off the shoulder and brachial plexus. For lung surgery the bed is often flexed to stretch out the ribs on the operative side; for kidney surgery the bed is flexed completely *and* the kidney rest is raised. Padding is placed beneath the lower leg and between the lower and upper legs. Long pieces of tape may be wrapped across the patient to keep him from rolling either forward or back, or a beanbag can be used. This wonderful device is soft and sandy when the patient first lies on it, and it can be molded up around the patient on either side. Then suction is applied, the sand is forcibly settled, and the thing takes on the consistency of concrete. The patient is thus secured in whatever position you want; just make sure you haven't left him or her

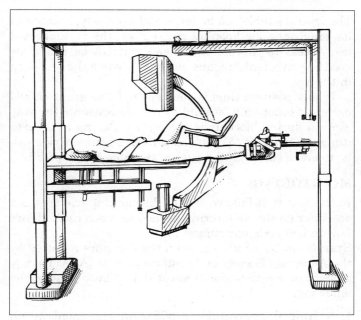

Fig. 1-9. The fracture table.

lying on an ECG lead when you do this. The lower arm is extended 90 degrees out in front of the patient, with liberal padding under the elbow and wrist. The upper arm can be stacked on top, with a pillow or two between, or suspended in an "airplane," an adjustable support that attaches to the bed. The latter device is recommended for cases where the position is "semi-lateral," with the patient's hips rolled back flat to allow an abdominal extension to the thoracic incision.

The **fracture table** (Fig. 1-9) is used to position a patient for open reduction and internal fixation of the hip. The patient is supine, with the affected leg in traction and the opposite leg lifted up into a medium-height stirrup. This allows the whole lower part of the table to be removed, so that a C-arm can be used to fluoroscope the hip during surgery. The contralateral arm is extended out on an armboard, but the ipsilateral arm is usually secured across the patient's chest. The bed is elevated toward the ceiling so that the surgeon can stand comfortably beside the patient and look straight at the hip.

The fracture table can be large and unwieldy, because of its provisions for keeping traction on the unsupported leg. Access to the patient's head will not be nearly as good as you might imagine, especially when the bed is up in the air.

In any position time is your enemy. The anesthetized patient cannot shift around to relieve bedsores the way *you* did during biochemistry lectures. During long cases it may be prudent to check on pressure points periodically, to make sure that the patient remains on the padding.

MONITORING

In the text that follows, one of the running features is a one-liner on the monitoring needed for each case. Here's how to translate our suggestions:

Standard: By which we mean the monitors required by the American Society of Anesthesiologists (ASA) for any general or major regional anesthetic. These include the following:

1. A trained anesthesia provider in the room at all times—you!
2. ECG
3. Pulse oximetry
4. Blood pressure, either automated or (gasp!) manual
5. Patient temperature measuring must be available.
6. Capnography is required for general anesthetics.
7. Measurement of FiO_2

We would also highly encourage a precordial or esophageal stethoscope and inspired and expired agent analysis, if available.

Foley Catheter: For relieving bladder distention in long cases and for closely following urine output in cases where fluid shifts or renal function are a concern.

Arterial Line (A-line): Used to follow blood pressure on a beat-to-beat basis in cases or patients where it is apt to change quickly. Also useful in patients who are going to need repeated lab draws for arterial blood gas (ABG), hematocrit, prothrombin time/partial thromboplastin time (PT/PTT), or electrolytes.

Pulmonary Artery (PA) Catheter: A PA, or Swan-Ganz, catheter is placed through a large-bore introducer from the internal jugular or subclavian artery, through the right atrium and right ventricle, and into a main pulmonary artery. The typical specimen will have lumens opening in the right atrium and at the tip for measurement of central venous pressure (CVP) and pulmonary artery pressure, respectively; a thermistor at the tip for measurement of blood temperature; and a balloon at the tip that, when inflated, will carry the distal tip into a "wedge" position in the pulmonary artery. When wedged, the distal port will be sealed off from pulmonary artery pressure by the balloon and will instead be looking at a fluid column extending forward into the left atrium. This pressure more or less (depending on cardiac valve function and the degree of pulmonary hypertension) corresponds to left ventricular preload. When hooked to a cardiac output machine, injection of fluid via the CVP port can be used to measure cardiac output. A venous infusion port (VIP) PA catheter has an extra lumen opening in the right atrium for central delivery of drug infusions. It is important to note that while the introducer for the PA catheter alone provides excellent large-bore vascular access, this capacity is diminished when the PA catheter is threaded through it.

TEE: Transesophageal echocardiography works via a really ugly looking probe that is inserted through the mouth and into the distal esophagus. Excellent images of the heart can be obtained in a variety of planes. The TEE is useful as a monitor for embolized air, as a means to assess cardiac valve function, and as an indicator of regional cardiac wall motion abnormalities. Unfortunately for us average schmoes, a TEE requires an experienced operator to generate and interpret the pictures.

Somatosensory Evoked Potentials (SSEP), Electroencephalogram (EEG), Peripheral Nerve Monitors, and Other Weirdness: These esoteric monitors each have specific uses in specific cases. See the text on each case for details.

BLOOD LOSS

Blood transfusions are presently given only to increase the patient's oxygen-carrying capacity. Blood also augments intravascular volume; however, this can be achieved with crystalloid and colloid without increasing the risk of infection or transfusion reaction. It is difficult to know at exactly what point a given individual requires transfusion, but it is inevitably based on multiple factors that include the patient's age, cardiovascular status, expected additional blood loss, starting hematocrit, and rate of ongoing blood loss. The National Institutes of Health (NIH) suggest that transfusions are not required for hemoglobin greater than 10 but frequently required for hemoglobin less than 7.

Type O-negative blood is the universal donor. In the uncommon circumstance when a patient receives greater than 2 units of type O-negative *whole blood* (rather than packed red blood cells) and requires additional transfusions, then recrossmatching is required prior to switching to the patient's original blood type. Type and screen (T&S) refers to determining the patient's ABO type and major red cell antigens. It is an alternative to crossmatch in situations where transfusion is less likely. If the T&S patient requires transfusion, a crossmatch must still be done. Type and crossmatch (T&C) involves selecting units that appear compatible based on the T&S and mixing a sample of the selected cells with the potential recipient's serum. If no agglutination or hemolysis occurs, the unit is deemed compatible. This specific unit is then set aside for this specific patient, removing it from the general blood bank supply.

Whole Blood: A typical unit is 450 ml and, if refrigerated for more than 24 hours, is devoid of platelet function. It contains all coagulation factors except V and VIII. Not usually available from most blood banks.

Packed Red Blood Cells (PRBCs): The usual volume is 250 ml and the hematocrit (HCT) is approximately 70%. They are derived from a unit of whole blood by centrifugation or sedimentation. Storage life is as great as 42 days if stored with Adsol, less than that with other agents.

Fresh-Frozen Plasma (FFP): The usual volume is 250 ml. It is produced from the centrifugation of a unit of whole blood that produces plasma, which in turn is cooled to −18°C within 6 hours. FFP can be stored for 1 year. The freezing preserves all coagulation factors including V and VIII. If not frozen, factor VIII declines 51% after 1 day of storage. Factor V declines more slowly. FFP also contains 500 mg of fibrinogen. FFP contains ABO isoagglutinins and must therefore be crossmatched for a particular patient.

Platelets: Each unit of platelets is prepared from a single unit of whole blood by centrifugation and resuspension in 50 ml of plasma. Each unit of transfused platelets should raise the platelet count by 5,000 to 10,000. ABO compatibility is desired but not required; there may be a small reduction in platelet survival if the unit is not ABO compatible. Remember that platelet count does not always correlate with bleeding. Platelets do not express Rh antigens. Platelet units do contain minimal red blood cell contamination, but this is insufficient to cause a hemolytic transfusion reaction.

Cryoprecipitate: Cryoprecipitate is produced by thawing a unit of FFP to 4°C. Total volume is 10–15 ml. Cryoprecipitate contains the procoagulant and platelet adhesive activities of factor VIII. It also contains fibrinogen (265 mg) and factor XIII. One unit of cryoprecipitate will raise the fibrinogen level about 5 mg/dl.

Never assume a patient's ABO group from previous records. Check blood products for correct type and crossmatch as soon as possible after they arrive in the OR. Return unused blood (and used paperwork) to the blood bank as soon as possible. When transfusing, you must at least verify the patient's name, ABO type, and unit number on both the patient record and the unit of blood issued by the blood bank, as well as checking the unit's expiration date. Use a filter when giving PRBCs or FFP. Filters (170–220 μm) remove microaggregates, which may otherwise clog the line or cause an immune reaction in the patient. Filters will clog up after several units of blood and should be changed periodically to maintain good flow.

Many components of the transfusion reaction are not detectable under general anesthesia. Acute hemolytic reactions can be accompanied by chills, fever, pain at the infusion site, substernal discomfort, dyspnea, and discomfort. The mechanism is interaction between recipient antibody and donor blood cells. Hypotension, renal failure, and vascular collapse are the extremes of the transfusion reaction. The treatment of transfusion reaction requires immediately stopping the transfusion, restoring blood pressure with fluids and vasopressors as indicated, and using diuretics (furosemide and mannitol) to maintain a brisk urine output. Additionally, a new blood sample should be drawn from the patient and sent for crossmatch. The risk of transfusing Rh-positive blood to an Rh-negative individual is not immediate hemolysis but sensitization of the patient (only a concern for a patient likely to become pregnant.) In the already sensitized patient, of course, a reaction will occur.

POSTOPERATIVE ANALGESIA

We believe, as we hope you do, that your job does not end when you drop the patient off in the postanesthesia care unit (PACU). Postoperative pain is caused by operative events, and postoperative pain management is best begun during the operative period. Knowing how much pain the patient will experience when the anesthetic wears off is an important part of your job, so for each surgery we review we give our recommendations for postoperative pain management. We've used a mildly cryptic system to categorize our observations, but don't despair! Here's the key:

Category I: No pain and no pain management required. This includes procedures such as MRI scans, cystoscopies, and bronchoscopies. The procedure itself might be quite stimulating, but no tissue is traumatized and nothing hurts postoperatively.

Category II: Minimal to moderate pain, usually relieved by oral analgesics like acetaminophen with codeine or codone (Tylenol No. 3, Percocet, or Tylox). This implies that the surgery is on a small scale and the intraoperative analgesia should last until the patient is able to take oral medications. One or two IM injections, typically ketorolac or meperidine, or a small dose of IV morphine may be needed to tide the patient over in the PACU. An even better strategy is to get the surgeon to infiltrate the skin and muscle incisions with local anesthesia during the closure; this will last longer than anything you can give parenterally and will be less sedating.

Category III: Moderate pain in a patient who may be NPO for several days. The traditional approach in this patient is serial IM doses of morphine or meperidine until the patient recovers enough to take oral medications. No one—patients or nurses—likes this approach very much, and technology has now brought us some alternatives. IV patient-controlled analgesia (PCA) attaches the patient's IV to a reservoir of narcotic, typically morphine, metered out by a computerized pump in response to the patient pushing a button. Psychologically, this puts the patient in the driver's seat. Not surprisingly, this system has been found to provide vastly superior analgesia and may even hasten patient recovery. The down side is that the analgesic is still administered parenterally and may cause sedation, respiratory depression, and a prolonged ileus.

Morphine may also be administered intrathecally, by itself or as part of a planned spinal anesthetic. This approach supplies excellent analgesia without a lot of systemic side effects but is limited by its finite duration (no more than 24 hours) and the need for careful respiratory monitoring. In some hospitals patients who have received intrathecal morphine can go straight from the PACU to the ward; in other hospitals they must remain 24 hours in a monitored setting.

Another option for the patient with category III pain is a continuous nonparenteral infusion administered via an epidural, caudal, or brachial plexus catheter. This infusion may be a local anesthetic alone (as in the brachial plexus) or an anesthetic combined with a low dose of narcotic (as in the epidural space). The infusion can be maintained as long as necessary and usually has minimal systemic and respiratory side effects. The down side, as with the single shot intrathecal narcotic, is that not all ward nurses are prepared to handle an epidural infusion. A set of standardized orders is probably the best and safest approach. Know your local policies!

Category IV: Serious pain, typically caused by an upper abdominal or thoracic incision that is continually irritated by breathing, coughing, moving, or displaying other signs of life. IV PCA will provide adequate analgesia for these patients, but the doses used will be high, and the accompanying sedation may inhibit coughing and deep breathing.

These are the patients to set up for a combined GETA/epidural anesthetic and a postoperative epidural infusion, if your local circumstances allow. A thoracic epidural will give you more bang for your buck, but a lumbar catheter will usually function just as well, with a slightly higher dose rate. With an epidural infusion in place these patients can be up and around on postoperative day one—ambulating, coughing, and deep breathing.

ANESTHETIC TECHNIQUES

One of the standard lines in our case-by-case descriptions is "acceptable techniques," by which we mean the more obvious choices for doing a given anesthetic—not all the choices, just the more common, more reasonable ones. If you want to do a mastectomy under a high spinal anesthetic, feel free—just don't expect us to staff you. Whatever anesthetic you choose must meet the goals of (1) patient safety, (2) facilitation of the surgery, and (3) patient comfort. Here's what we mean by what we recommend:

None: The procedure can be done without anesthesia at all—MRI scans or vaginal deliveries, for example. Your help is not required.

Local: The surgeon injects local anesthesia into the area of surgery, then operates on it. Once again, your participation is unnecessary.

MAC: Monitored anesthesia care. You are now involved. Your job is, as always, to keep the patient alive and comfortable throughout the procedure. This may consist of no more than hand holding, while the surgeon works on an area blocked by local anesthesia, or IV sedation ranging from minimal to near general anesthesia. Titration to the needs of the patient is very important, as is the ability to recognize when to pull the plug and convert to a general anesthetic.

GA: General anesthesia; when expressed this way, it means you have a choice of whether or not to intubate the patient. This designation usually appears on short cases where the upper body, head, or neck is not involved. General anesthesia implies ASA standard monitoring (see the section on monitoring) and postoperative recovery in the PACU.

GETA: General endotracheal anesthesia, meaning that intubation is likely to be necessary, because of the area being operated on, the length of the surgery, or the need for positive pressure ventilation.

Spinal: Most useful for surgeries below the diaphragm. Advantages include ease of administration, rapid onset, and predictable level. Disadvantages include limited duration, (which can be up to 8 hours if the right local anesthetic is chosen, but the decision has to be made up front); rapid onset, which may cause rapid hemodynamic shifts; and incomplete anesthesia of the peritoneum, which makes it a bad choice for surgeries where the patient is not highly motivated to remain awake.

Epidural: Useful for the same range of surgeries that a spinal is. Advantages include the ability to bring the level up more slowly (conferring greater hemodynamic stability), the ability to redose the catheter if the procedure lasts longer than expected, and the ability to leave the catheter in for postoperative analgesia. Disadvantages are a more complicated procedure, a bigger needle, slower onset of anesthesia, and a less intense block, particularly in the distal lower extremities and upper abdomen. The risk of a postdural puncture headache is about the same with an epidural (where dural puncture is inadvertent but very likely to produce a headache) and a spinal (where dural puncture is deliberate but small enough to cause a headache only infrequently). The risk of an epidural hematoma may be greater with an epidural, because the needle size is larger.

Combined: Refers in this text to the use of a regional anesthetic, typically an epidural, with a light GETA. The former supplies the bulk of the anesthesia and a good start on postoperative analgesia. The latter allows for positive pressure ventilation and control of stimulation outside the coverage of the epidural. This technique is typically used for hemodynamically tenuous patients or those with an anticipated large postoperative analgesic requirement.

Ankle Block, Leg Block, Axillary Block, Interscalene Block: Various regional procedures designed to numb just one portion of the body. Unlike epidurals and spinals, a large volume of local anesthetic is used, which can cause toxic complications. On the other hand, once the block is in and working, it will last for 6–8 hours without further maintenance. This makes them good for postoperative analgesia as well. For longer, bigger cases the block can be combined with a general anesthetic.

Bier Block: A strange fish in the sea of regional anesthetics. Administered IV, the block is good for only 60–90 minutes. This technique is most useful for short hand or foot cases where the patient and surgeon desire a speedy resolution of the block. Toxic complications are likely if the tourniquet is released within the first half hour.

OPERATING ROOM SET-UP

We know we can't possibly predict every piece of equipment you might want in the OR for a particular case, although we have taken pains to tell you what we can. The following list should therefore be construed as no more than a bare minimum, for a generic simple case. You can make up your own mnemonic—the one we use is not suitable for print.

I. Suction
Working pharyngeal suction tubing (Yankauer) and endotracheal suction catheters

II. Monitors
Noninvasive blood pressure, with appropriately sized cuff

Pulse oximeter, with appropriate probe

Temperature probe and monitor

ECG with five-lead cable

Precordial or esophageal stethoscope

Nerve stimulator

FiO_2 monitor, calibrated

CO_2 monitor, calibrated

III. Drugs—Have these things drawn up:
Sodium thiopental—2×500 mg (can substitute propofol or etomidate)

Succinylcholine—200 mg

Nondepolarizing relaxant—dealer's choice. Because these tend to be expensive agents, you may only want to draw them up when you know you're going to use them.
Ephedrine—50 mg
Epinephrine—1 mg
Atropine—1 mg
Lidocaine—100 mg

The last three items may exist as prepackaged syringes that you can check once, throw in your bag, and have ready whenever you need them.

IV. Airway stuff
Face mask, multiple sizes
Oral and nasal airways, in appropriate sizes
Anesthesia circuit
Endotracheal tubes—6.0, 7.0, 7.5, 8.0 sizes—with cuff syringes
Laryngoscope handle, two
Laryngoscope blades, Miller No. 2, No. 3 and Macintosh No. 3, No. 4
"Tube tree" (that nasty metal thing that holds up the circuit)
V. Miscellaneous stuff
ECG pads
Nasogastric tube
Lots of syringes and needles
IV hardware
Lactated Ringer's, lots
Normal saline
Tape, in a variety of sizes and types

TEMPERATURE

Throughout the rest of this book, whenever you are reading about a large case, you will see the occasional cryptic reminder to "keep the patient warm." We now explain what we mean by that.

Patients get cold for a variety of reasons: loss of fluid from the respiratory tract due to breathing dry gases (evaporation); transfer of heat to the operating table (conduction); heat loss to cold room air (convection); and "black body" loss to the environment (radiation). Heat loss also occurs, via convection and evaporation, from exposed tissue like the gut. Anesthesia worsens heat loss by preventing shivering, altering thermoregulation, and dilating peripheral vessels. Elderly patients cool even faster than young adults because of lower metabolic rates, impaired thermoregulatory systems, and decreased autonomic control. Pediatric patients cool quickly because of their high body surface to mass ratio. Cold IV infusions are a major contributor.

Hypothermia is bad for a variety of reasons. Anesthetic drug elimination is slowed, which may delay awakening. Neuromuscular blockade may be prolonged. Oxygen delivery is decreased, and coagulation and platelet function may be impaired. Renal blood flow is decreased and peripheral perfusion suffers. Extreme hypothermia (around 30°C) will lead to bradycardia, atrial fibrillation, ventricular fibrillation, and asystole. Even mild hypothermia is bad because it builds up a metabolic debt the patient will have to repay in the PACU. Postoperative shivering raises the basal metabolic rate and increases oxygen consumption, thereby straining the cardiovascular system. Cold may even depress respiratory drive, especially in neonates, which will further delay emergence.

So, how does one warm a patient in the OR? The best way is to anticipate the problem and keep the patient from ever getting cold. This can be done by keeping the ambient temperature up and the patient well insulated. Wrap the head and unused body parts in warm blankets or plastic and keep the room temperature as high as the surgeons will tolerate.

Fluids going into the patient should be warmed, and several devices exist for administering large volumes of warmed fluids quickly. (We like the Level One infuser.) Warming blood and blood products is an especially good idea, since they usually start out much colder than room temperature.

Heat loss to evaporation can be prevented by using any one of many humidifying devices designed to keep moisture in the lungs. Active warming and humidification of gases is recommended for big cases and can actually warm up an already cold patient. Make sure the active heater's airway temperature probe is appropriately installed near the Y in your circuit, or you may accidentally overdo it.

Irrigation fluid should be warm, especially in the peritoneum or chest. If the patient is cold the irrigation can be repeated several times and may actually help warm the patient.

A warming blanket can be placed on the bed and will prevent some conductive heat loss. As an active warming device, however, it is just about useless. If not adequately padded, it can be downright uncomfortable. More useful are the new generation of warm air (convection) blankets, which are very effective in warming hypothermic patients.

Warming lights ("French fry lights") are good only if your patient is smaller than a bread box. In adult patients they mostly just get in the way. If used improperly they can cause significant skin burns.

Turn the room temperature up. Did we mention that one already? Heat is easy to lose and hard to get back. Plan ahead.

TRAUMA

When dealing with the acutely traumatized patient, remember the ABCs:

A is for Airway: Securing it safely is your biggest challenge. All trauma patients have full stomachs and are at high risk for aspiration. Many will have stomachs full of alcohol, which will increase their risk even further. Consider administering prophylactic H_2-blockers or a nonparticulate antacid.

Consider the possibility of a cervical spine injury before rushing to intubate the patient. If the airway does need to be secured in a hurry, anesthetize or paralyze the patient as needed and intubate orally with a laryngoscope. Have an assistant provide in-line cervical traction to the head and neck.

Nasotracheal intubation is contraindicated in the presence of a suspected cribriform plate fracture or obvious facial trauma.

Lidocaine (100 mg IV) given just prior to laryngoscopy will help minimize rises in intracranial pressure (ICP).

Traditional induction agents may be contraindicated by extreme volume depletion. Consider using fentanyl, etomidate, or ketamine.

Evidence of possible tracheal or laryngeal damage includes hoarseness, stridor, and subcutaneous emphysema; if present, these signs should be a warning to approach the airway cautiously.

The nasogastric tube, if already present, should either be removed or left open to air when intubating to provide a channel for relieving gastric pressure during induction. If not already present, leave it out until after the tube is in.

B is for Breathing: Start with 100% oxygen and work down from there. Suspect a pneumothorax at all times, and be prepared to treat it aggressively.

The lungs can be contused by blunt trauma, making the patient prone to pulmonary edema and hypoxia. Treat with an elevated FiO_2 and positive end-expiratory pressure (PEEP) (which may decrease cardiac output), and try not to overdo the fluid resuscitation (difficult in a trauma patient). Give furosemide early.

Air in places it shouldn't be (like a pneumothorax) will expand in the presence of nitrous oxide. Don't use nitrous until you're sure it's OK.

C is for Circulation: Get yourself plenty of large-bore IV access early in the proceedings. Two 14-gauge antecubital catheters are standard for trauma resuscitation.

An arterial line will be a must for any major trauma, but it may have to wait until after induction.

Blunt chest trauma may lead to cardiac contusion, pericardial tamponade, or dissection of the aorta. Suspect these things, along with continued occult blood loss, if the patient is not responding appropriately to volume loading.

Stick with nonvasodilating agents (like fentanyl) until you know the blood loss is under control. Make the patient ask for the isoflurane. Don't be surprised if your anesthetic consists of no more than muscle relaxants and oxygen, especially early in the case. And don't worry—hypotension and closed head trauma are excellent amnestics. Give a little scopolomine (0.2 mg IV) if you're worried about recall.

Crystalloid solutions will rapidly equilibrate with the extravascular space. Colloids will provide a more sustained resuscitation, at the possible risk of greater edema later on.

Dilutional coagulopathies are common when blood loss is high. Think about FFP after 6–8 units of PRBCs, if a substantial amount of further bleeding is anticipated, and plan on 1 unit of FFP for each unit of PRBC thereafter. Platelets will become necessary after about 10 units of PRBCs and regularly thereafter at a rate of about 1 unit per unit. Guide your therapy by specific studies (HCT, platelet count, PT/PTT) whenever possible, but don't hesitate to treat empirically if it looks like the patient is going down the tubes.

Large transfusions also lead to a need for calcium and bicarbonate. Use an ABG and ionized calcium measurement to guide you.

D is for Etc.: Make sure someone has done a thorough secondary assessment before getting too obsessed with repairing things. Missing a ruptured spleen when you're doing an orthopedic case (for example) can lead to a really nasty intraoperative surprise.

Keep the patient warm from the start. Warm the OR, warm all the fluids, and cover up what the surgeons aren't working on.

Extubation can await a later day, when cardiac and pulmonary contusions have resolved and perioperative fluid shifts have passed. Err on the side of keeping the patient intubated.

Get help early and keep it late. If nothing else you will need extra hands to hang or squeeze blood, but additional bodies can also be put to work on obtaining extra access, keeping the paperwork straight, running blood gases, or hand-ventilating the patient.

Be careful when transferring the patient to the ICU. Losing lines during a move can ultimately prove lethal. Make sure you have resuscitation drugs and equipment for reintubating along with you (a pain in the neck until the day you need them).

PEDIATRICS

Yes, we know we have a chapter on pediatric surgery elsewhere in this book, but kids do the darndest things, and not all of the possible operations are in that chapter.

This section provides a quick and dirty guide to anesthetizing children, with material applicable to any case.

First of all, plan on a general anesthetic. Kids won't hold still for a regional and won't hold still once it's in. Once they're asleep, however, you can sneak your regional analgesic in, whether a caudal, an epidural, or a field block. Regional *is* the best approach for postoperative analgesia.

Getting the patient asleep can be a problem as well. If the child is NPO you have a relatively easy chore and a lot of options. You can begin with oral or nasal midazolam, rectal methohexital, or a lot of sweet talk to get the child away from Mom, then breathe them down in the OR, start their IV, intubate (if necessary), and let the surgeon get started.

In the child with a full stomach or some other reason to be concerned about aspiration, your options are considerably less pleasant. Someone—meaning you—is going to have to hold the child down and start an IV before you can induce anesthesia. Once the IV is in, the rest of your day should be easy, since kids mostly have good hearts and straightforward airways and respond consistently to drugs given on a per-kilogram basis (once they've grown out of the neonatal period, that is).

Things to have handy when approaching a pediatric case:

1. Appropriate monitoring equipment, including the right size blood pressure cuff and oximeter probe
2. Pediatric laryngoscope blades in a variety of sizes and styles
3. A range of small endotracheal tubes, masks, and oral airways
4. 22- and 24-gauge IVs
5. A de-aired IV setup incorporating a calibrated drip chamber (Buretrol) so you can follow infused fluids closely
6. Warming lights for the really small kids.

Drugs to have ready include thiopental, succinylcholine, atropine, and your favorite muscle relaxant. Draw them up in small syringes, to a specific mg/kg dose, so that if you need them you're all ready to go. Remember that in pediatric patients stroke volume is fixed, and cardiac output depends on heart rate. Atropine is your friend in almost any crisis; give it early.

Needless to say (but we'll say it anyway), pediatric patients get cold a lot faster than adults. Keep the room temperature up, and keep the patient covered whenever possible. Also follow fluids closely, since the kid's circulating volume is small. Both exsanguination and fluid overload are easy to achieve.

Most pediatric patients can be easily extubated at the end of the procedure, but you will still need to pay close attention. Children have a higher metabolic rate and a lower functional residual capacity (FRC) than adults, meaning that they will desaturate a lot faster when the airway is obstructed. Kids are also quite prone to laryngospasm, which can darken anyone's day. We like to keep a unit dose of succinylcholine (4 mg/kg) and atropine (0.1 mg/kg) on hand for IM injection in case of an airway crisis.

Postoperatively, children are more likely to be fussy because they are hungry and in a strange place than because they are in pain. Try to get some local anesthetic into every pediatric surgical patient, even if you just have the surgeon splash some bupivacaine in the wound during closure. Then you can treat your fussy patient in the PACU with a little PO or rectal acetaminophen, which has an amazingly good effect, and avoid any use of narcotics. When psychosocial issues seem prominent, let the parents come in. Often the presence of Mom and Dad will make all the difference.

Bradycardia equals hypoxemia, until proven otherwise.

THE PREGNANT PATIENT

One of the scariest things that can happen to you in the OR is to get assigned to anesthetize a pregnant patient for nonobstetric surgery. The stakes are doubled, as it were, and you suddenly have a large number of physiologic concerns you didn't have before. But have no fear, we're here to help. (You can trust us, we're from the government.)

First of all, read the chapter introduction for obstetric anesthesia, which summarizes the physiologic changes of pregnancy. Then come back here for a few specific comments.

All elective surgery should be postponed until after delivery. The risks of teratogenesis and/or preterm labor are just too high, even for simple cases that would normally be no big deal. This means that the case you are confronted with will be urgent at the very least (like a hot gallbladder or appendix) or possibly even emergent (trauma of some kind).

Get your obstetric colleagues involved early and make them take a stand on whether the fetus is likely to be viable or not. This is important both for determining how aggressively to monitor fetal heart tones and for how to present the risks of anesthesia and surgery to the mother. If the child is likely to be viable, then continuous fetal heart rate (FHR) monitoring is recommended, prophylactic tocolysis may be in order (check with the obstetrician), and everyone involved should be prepared for an emergency C-section. If the fetus is judged to be too immature to survive, then FHR monitoring should occur before and after surgery (for documentation purposes) and the mother should be counseled specifically about the risk of a miscarriage.

In late pregnancy it becomes important for you to avoid fetal asphyxia, which means maintaining a maximal delivery of oxygen to the placenta. Keep Mom's blood pressure up by maintaining left uterine displacement and minimizing aortocaval compression (Fig. 1-10), keep Mom's blood well saturated with oxygen, keep the uterus from contracting, and avoid things that increase Mom's catecholamine level. Neither regional nor general anesthesia maintains uterine blood flow better than the other. Regional has the advantage of involving fewer potentially harmful agents. General has the advantage (in the case of volatile anesthetics) of blocking uterine contractions.

As far as teratogenicity goes, the bottom line is that few data have been accumulated in humans. Benzodiazepines have been associated with an increased incidence of cleft palate deformities, spina bifida, and possibly cardiac anomalies and therefore should be avoided. Nitrous oxide is known to inhibit methionine synthetase

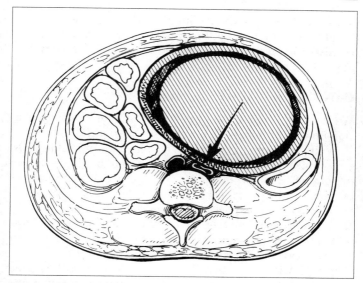

Fig. 1-10. Aortocaval compression.

production, and hence DNA development, in the laboratory. No adverse outcome with N_2O has been documented in humans, but most practitioners prefer to avoid its use. That covers the known bad actors.

Volatile anesthetics are probably safe and are tocolytic. Narcotics are probably safe, but will also narcotize the fetus (causing decreased respiration if delivered and decreased FHR variability). Muscle relaxants are probably safe because they do not cross the placenta very well. Local anesthetics are probably safe but may cause neurobehavioral changes in an infant delivered soon after their administration. Ditto for thiopental, propofol, etomidate, and ketamine. In other words, nothing is known about the potential of these agents for causing birth defects, but we do know that if you deliver a baby when the mother is under general anesthesia, the baby will generally be anesthetized as well, depending on how long it takes to go from induction to delivery.

So, in summary: tip the patient to the left, avoid aspiration and airway difficulties by doing a regional anesthetic, use lower doses of drugs, use short-acting agents, avoid nitrous oxide and benzodiazepines, maintain maternal blood pressure, and counsel the patient before-hand about the risks of birth defects and preterm labor. Involve the obstetricians from the start. Cross your fingers.

CANCER SURGERY

We hear you asking the question: "Why a separate section on cancer surgery? What's the big deal?"

Well, try putting yourself in the patient's place. Do you think you'd be feeling better about having a lower abdominal incision for delivery of your child or removal of your ovarian cancer? We'd rather have the baby, thanks, and we expect you would too. The most important difference between benign operations and those where cancer is a concern is patient anxiety. Expect the patient to be hospital-wise and to ask many questions. Not only will patients with cancer or suspected cancer typically require a great deal more premedication than patients who know their disease is benign, but they also will require more postoperative analgesia as well. Don't believe us? Take a look through your PACU some day and compare the patients who had mastectomies for cancer with those who had plastic surgery breast reductions.

Your approach to the cancer patient will be different as well. Joking is fine with the 20-year-old having a knee operation because he skis too hard, but believe us, neither of you will feel like joking when you meet the same patient with an osteosarcoma.

Cancer patients may have had multiple previous operations, and may look very ill. IV access will be difficult, and the patient may tolerate your attempts poorly. "Hospitalitis" has set in. Our advice is to look for the central line early.

Once you make it into the OR you will still have some things to consider. The patient will most likely want to go to sleep, and you should most likely oblige. Once induced, the psychological factors diminish, but the anatomic ones remain. The operation may become much longer than anticipated if an invasive cancer is discovered, or much shorter if the patient's disease is deemed inoperable. There may be waiting periods for pathology reports. Dissection may be interminable, if an en bloc resection is elected. Complications can arise from trying to pry the cancer off vessels or nerves.

Patients who have had chemotherapy or radiation may also give you trouble. Adriamycin administration permanently damages the heart, as manifested by a decreased ejection fraction; bleomycin can cause restrictive lung physiology, which may be exacerbated by high concentrations of oxygen; and steroid administration may produce adrenal suppression, necessitating stress doses of steroids perioperatively. Radiation, meanwhile, can directly damage the lungs, heart, and bone marrow, and will produce scarring and fibrosis at the surgical site.

You should be prepared with plenty of access, plenty of warm fluids, plenty of compassion, and plenty of patience. Be generous with your anesthetic and analgesics, and take the case as seriously as the patient does.

LAPAROSCOPY

... means never having to say atelectasis. This newfangled technique has caught on rapidly in the last decade because of the associated reduction in postoperative pain, hospital stay, recovery time, and $$$. General surgeons and gynecologists use laparoscopy routinely for resection of the gallbladder, ovary, appendix, and colon, and for assessing fallopian tube function, assisting in dissection of the uterus, taking down adhesions, repairing hernias—both hiatal and inguinal—and simply looking around. The few small incisions associated with a laparoscopy cause minimal disruption of the abdominal musculature and allow the patient to make a fast and relatively pain-free recovery. Consider these points when planning for a laparoscopy case:

In order to see anything, the surgeon must expand the peritoneum with a pressurized gas, typically CO_2. This abdominal distension makes the procedure stimulating while it is underway and almost mandates a general anesthetic. Upward pressure on the diaphragm will decrease pulmonary compliance, while absorption of CO_2 will create a mild acidemia. We usually ignore the rise in end-tidal CO_2, as long as oxygenation remains adequate.

A Foley catheter will be required to make the bladder a smaller target for percutaneous trocar placement. Ditto with an orogastric tube and the stomach.

A regional anesthetic will require a high level and a very motivated patient. Nausea and vague discomfort from peritoneal traction are common.

The surgeon will probably ask for the bed to be tipped toward the feet (if operating in the upper abdomen) or head (if operating in the pelvis) to better view the area of interest. Either way this will have an effect on ventilation and blood pressure that you should be expecting.

Vagal responses—including asystole—are not uncommon with peritoneal distension. Having the patient deep enough to avoid reflex responses will help dodge this problem, as will the liberal use of atropine at the first sign of trouble.

Other disastrous complications are caused by misplacement of the insufflating trocar. Hitting the aorta will be immediately apparent. Hitting a large vein will lead to a CO_2 embolus that can be life threatening. Hitting the gut will cause contamination of the peritoneum and abdominal wall and the cessation of the procedure. Hitting the bladder can occur but is generally avoided by placing a Foley catheter first to decompress it. Falling short of the abdominal wall will lead to insufflation between muscle layers, which is confusing to the surgeon but not life threatening to the patient. Nicking a small vessel in the peritoneum or retroperitoneum may cause an occult bleeding problem that only becomes apparent hours later. The solution to most of these errors is an immediate laparotomy, which the patient should have been counseled about.

Finally, the use of nitrous oxide during laparoscopy is somewhat controversial. In most cases it is no big deal, but in longer or more difficult procedures it may cause sufficient distension of the gut to obscure the surgeon's view.

There is also a (theoretical) concern with nitrous being able to support combustion. The combination of methane from the gut, nitrous oxide diffused into gut and peritoneum, and a spark from the electrocautery has been shown to be explosive in the laboratory. (What a great research project: "I'm going to be a little late today,

honey; I'm going over to the lab to blow up a few pigs.")
To date there have been no case reports of exploding
patients, although someday someone is going to be the
first. Current recommendations call for turning off the
nitrous if the integrity of the gut is violated.

OBESITY

When faced with patients who are significantly short of
their ideal body height, you will have many opportunities
for excitement. Everything you do, everything the nurses do, and everything the surgeon does will be harder.
Here are some tips for survival:

1. Be up-front about the difficulties you will encounter. Most of these patients realize they are overweight
and will appreciate an honest description of what's going
to happen to them.

2. Allow extra time for getting your lines in place. IVs
may be difficult, and it won't help anything if you're feeling rushed. Central lines in the neck may be harder; subclavian and antecubital lines are usually not too bad.

3. Obese patients are at high risk for aspiration.
Prophylaxis is highly recommended, and awake or rapid-
sequence inductions are *de rigeur*.

4. Titration of many agents may be harder in obese
patients. The distinction between actual weight and lean
body mass may become relevant when predicting induction doses, and the fat solubility of some agents may
change their effective clearance in this population.

5. Lean toward a regional anesthetic. Surprisingly, the
epidural and intrathecal spaces are usually not too hard to
access. Keeping patients awake and breathing under their
own power will be enormously beneficial, and an epidural
can be continued into the postoperative period. If you must
do a general anesthetic, place the epidural catheter anyway and do a combined technique. You'll have the catheter
for postop pain, respiratory function will be improved, and
you'll be able to wake the patient quicker (after giving less
general anesthesia) and extubate earlier.

Take a good look at the airway before doing anything
stupid. Sometimes jowly patients have good mobility of

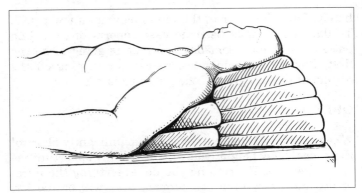

Fig. 1-11. One method for building up the shoulder and head to achieve a good sniffing position in the morbidly obese patient.

their necks and can be easily intubated despite looking scary. Other times, though, intubation will be a problem. Don't hesitate to go the awake fiberoptic route if necessary. Figure 1–11 illustrates one method for building up the shoulders and head to achieve a good sniffing position in the massively obese patient.

Titrate your induction drugs carefully, rather than blasting them in. Fat is vessel-poor, so that giving an appropriate per-kilogram dose of thiopental to someone with a lot of fat can amount to a big overdose.

Position the patient carefully. Make sure the OR table is big enough for the job, and that you don't allow it to tip over. Pad under the patient carefully; more weight means more pressure on all the usual "pressure points."

Before extubating, pause for a moment to ask yourself if you are sure you will be able to reintubate if you have to. Make sure the patient is well awake. Sit him or her up as soon as the tube is out; this "positional panniculectomy" will greatly reduce the work of breathing.

LASERS

Lasers are one of those occupational hazards you will occasionally run into, even in the nicest of ORs. They may be used in plastic, ENT, thoracic, general, pediatric, neuro, urology, or gynecology cases, so there's no telling when you'll encounter your first laser case. Rather than panicking, just check out these important tips:

Lasers come in four basic types (at least right now): argon, CO_2, YAG, and "tunable gas." Although their wavelengths and safety concerns vary somewhat, they all do essentially the same thing: create a very tight, very powerful beam of energy. This beam can be used to destroy tissue, coagulate bleeding vessels, or both. Argon and gas lasers work in the visible spectrum, with a beam you can see; CO_2 and YAG lasers work in the infrared and are invisible but are often accompanied by a red light laser so you can see where they're aimed.

Lasers are great for destroying tissue that you want destroyed, but they suffer from a lack of discrimination. Reflections off shiny metal instruments can send beams almost anywhere, putting everyone in the room at risk. Skin burns are small, rare, and no big deal. Eye burns are another matter: CO_2 lasers can scar the cornea, whereas the other lasers can burn the retina directly. Everyone in the room must wear the appropriate eye protection as long as the laser is on. Glasses are clear for the CO_2 and YAG lasers (make sure you get the right pair!) and colored for the visible spectrum ones.

Make sure to cover the patient's eyes, as well, with a thick piece of gauze. If you are using the laser in the airway, you will also want to make sure you have minimized the risk of igniting your endotracheal tube: Use as little oxygen in air as you can get away with, and use an endotracheal tube specifically designed to be fire resistant (metal wrapped or silicon coated). Put saline in the endotracheal tube cuff instead of air, and have an additional supply of saline on hand to douse fires. If a fire does occur, turn off the gas, remove the burning endotracheal tube at once, and reintubate. Rigid bronchoscopy will be needed to assess the damage.

Finally, lasers require careful maintenance and must be specifically set up and calibrated for each case. Expect your room turnover to take a little longer while this is happening. Lasers also draw a lot of power and can set off circuit breakers in your monitoring equipment if your OR electrical system is not up to the challenge. Try and plug the laser in as far away from your machine as possible.

REFERENCES

We realize that there may be a few things about anesthesia that we're not telling you here, and we're tough enough to admit it. When you overcome the day-to-day challenges of clinical existence and want to learn a little more of the science behind our clinical recommendations, check out the following selections:

All-Purpose

Clinical Anesthesia, edited by Barash and Stoelting, has provided new competition for *Anesthesia*, edited by Miller, as the definitive big fat reference tome.

Clinical Anesthesia Procedures of the Massachusetts General Hospital, edited by Davison, Eckhardt, and Perese, is probably the most popular tote-around reference. The handbook version of Barash is OK too.

Anesthesia and Coexisting Disease, by Stoelting and Dierdorf, and *Anesthesia and Uncommon Diseases*, by Katz, Benumof, and Kadis, are the reference books we head for when we encounter an obscure medical problem. The former work is now out in handbook form, as well.

Obstetrics

Anesthesia for Obstetrics, edited by Shnider and Levinson, is a superb treatment of most obstetric anesthesia issues. *Anesthesia and Obstetric Management of High Risk Pregnancy*, edited by Datta, is also very good.

Cardiac

The Practice of Cardiac Anesthesia, by Hensley and Martin, is the best handbook to tote around and makes a useful read-through during your cardiac time. The best tome for the hardcore is Kaplan's *Cardiac Anesthesia*.

Thoracic

We like *Thoracic Anesthesia*, also edited by Kaplan. There is no good handbook on this topic, although the two general purpose handbooks referenced above both have chapters on thoracic anesthesia. (We prefer the one in the *Massachusetts General Hospital Handbook*, for obvious reasons.)

Regional

Techniques of Regional Anesthesia, by Scott, is a good handy reference. *Neural Blockade in Clinical Anesthesia and Management of Pain*, edited by Cousins, et al., is the definitive tome.

Pediatrics

A Practice of Anesthesia for Infants and Children by Cote, et al., is easy to read, is clinically oriented, and has a good selection of pictures and graphs.

Pain

The bible is Bonica's *Management of Pain*. We have yet to see a handbook that tells us what we need to know, but we keep loping. *Principles and Practice of Pain Management*, edited by Warfield, is a useful quick and dirty reference but is not small enough to easily tote around.

Neuro

The preferred handbook is *Neuroanesthesia: Handbook of Clinical and Physiologic Essentials* by Newfield and Cotrell. *Clinical Neuroanesthesia*, edited by Cucchiara and Michenfelder, is a more comprehensive (and less portable) reference.

Vascular

We like *Anesthesia for Vascular Surgery*, edited by Roizen, because it's up to the minute, handles the controversies well, and is easy to read.

Oral Boards

Read *Preparing for the Anesthesia Orals: Board Stiff*, by Gallagher and Lubarsky. Read it again. Read it on the airplane, read it in bed the night before the test. Not only does it tell you most of what you need to know about the orals and explain how to study for them, but it's also funny and easy to read. These guys are our idols, and we hope to join them on the beach someday.

General Surgery

As you will see from the rest of this chapter, general surgery can include almost anything, from lymph node biopsies anywhere in the body to day-long expeditions to the deepest reaches of the pelvis. Indeed, in a small hospital the general surgeon will do the work of half a dozen different specialties: colorectal, thoracic, vascular, and trauma surgery; urology; gynecology; orthopedics; gastroenterology; and so forth. For the purposes of this chapter, though, we have included only the more traditional cases of the general surgeon. A few of the cases listed in this chapter also appear elsewhere in this book, reflecting the considerable overlap that general surgeons have with other specialties.

General surgery patients can be big or small, old or young, healthy or sick. Operations are performed on both inpatients and outpatients. If you went into anesthesia for the variety of patients and problems you get to see, then general surgery would be a good choice if you ever decided to switch specialties. (Of course, all that variety comes with a price. The general surgery residency is at least 5 grueling years long. We recommend staying with anesthesia.)

The most common venue for the general surgeon is within the peritoneum. Operations on the gut make up the bulk of their business, and anesthesia for intra-abdominal surgery involves a few specific concerns. Third-space loss of fluid and heat can be substantial and can put a patient in the hurt locker if you're not paying adequate attention. Bleeding can be an insidious problem in the lower abdomen and an overwhelming concern in the upper part. Postoperative pain is usually severe, often requiring the most complex modalities you have to offer.

General surgery patients frequently have cancer, or are worried that they do. This anxiety leads to a whole separate set of concerns, which are summarized in the section on cancer surgery in Chapter 1.

General surgeons are also the biggest users of the laparoscope and will become more so as skills and equip-

ment improve. Specific concerns for laparoscopy are summarized in Chapter 1 and apply to many of the cases
here.

Finally, general surgeons do a lot of emergency cases.
From appendectomies to perforated ulcers, the general
surgeon is the one who gets to clean up after
humankind's more dramatic internal disasters. General
surgeons are also in charge of most trauma patients who
come to the OR and will be dealing with the most immediately life-threatening problems.

Upper Endoscopy

Description: The surgeons stick a very large fiberoptic scope down the patient's throat and examine the esophagus, the stomach, and the first part of the duodenum. Various devices can be introduced through the 'scope to give injections, cauterize tissue, or take biopsy samples.

Position:	Lateral "park bench"
Estimated time:	60 minutes
Estimated blood loss:	Zero
Need for muscle relaxation:	None
Indicated monitors:	Standard
Postoperative analgesia:	I; nothing
Acceptable techniques:	Usually local plus IV sedation

Comments: Only the sicker patients will tend to come to your attention, since the majority of these procedures are done in the clinic or outpatient center without your involvement. The patients you get to monitor will be bleeding heavily from their esophageal varices, be an ASA IV from their heart condition, be afflicted with senile dementia, or all three.

Pay attention to the surgeon as the upper airway is topicalized. You might learn something.

Beware of oversedating. Once the topicalization hits, there really isn't much stimulation provided by the procedure. Make sure you are providing supplemental oxygen, and take your monitoring seriously.

Futzing around in the lower esophagus can irritate the next organ forward, which is the heart. Beware of sudden arrhythmias.

Dread complications of perforating the stomach or esophagus include pneumothorax, infection, severe bleeding, and—usually—emergency surgery. Pay close attention to what your surgeon is biopsying.

Neck Biopsy

Description: The surgeon opens the superficial tissue of the neck, locates whatever lump is sought after, and removes it. This should be a simple case.

Position:	Supine, head turned
Estimated time:	60 minutes
Estimated blood loss:	Minimal
Need for muscle relaxation:	None
Indicated monitors:	Standard
Postoperative analgesia:	II; PO medications
Acceptable techniques:	Local, deep, and superficial cervical plexus block, GETA

Comments: Patients may be very nervous about their diagnosis and may consume large quantities of sedation.

This procedure is often done by junior surgical residents, which may make the dissection tedious.

Although it's rare to see a major mistake, the neck is high-value real estate. Accidental surgical entry into the trachea, carotid, jugular, pleura, or brachial plexus can all be disastrous. A postoperative hematoma can compromise the airway very quickly.

You probably won't have great access to the patient's face if things go wrong. Remember this before oversedating.

Hemorrhoidectomy/Anal Fistula Repair

Description: For a hemorrhoidectomy the surgeon simply exposes and ligates the offending vessels. For a fistula repair, the surgeon usually tries to open and drain the fistulous tract. Frankly, we've never been interested in taking a closer look.

Position:	Lithotomy or prone/jackknife
Estimated time:	60 minutes
Estimated blood loss:	Minimal
Need for muscle relaxation:	None
Indicated monitors:	Standard
Postoperative analgesia:	II; PO medications
Acceptable techniques:	GA, spinal, local

Comments: Local with sedation is fairly uncomfortable for the patient and can only be recommended for very short, very simple cases. Infected areas with a low tissue pH (abscesses) may not absorb local anesthetics very well.

The lithotomy position is great for mask general anesthesia, GETA, hyperbaric spinals, and short cases that become longer. The surgeons are a long way away and you have good access to the airway.

The prone position makes general anesthesia a pain in the butt (sorry) and IV sedation risky, but it's great for doing a hypobaric spinal. Get the patient to position himself comfortably first, crank a little Trendelenburg on, and go ahead and place the spinal needle with the patient jackknifed and head down (it's surprisingly easy). Then administer 5 ml of sterile water with 10 mg of tetracaine in it. A nice perineal block will form, the patient will be awake and comfortable, and you'll look like a star.

Inguinal Hernia

Description: The surgeon makes an incision in the crease of the groin, dissects out the hernia sac and the normal spermatic cord structures (in a male), ligates the former (sparing the latter), and cinches things closed again. If the normal structures for cinching are inadequate, then a piece of Marlex mesh is flopped over the hole and tacked down around the edges.

Position:	Supine
Estimated time:	90 minutes
Estimated blood loss:	Minimal
Need for muscle relaxation:	Helpful for closure
Indicated monitors:	Standard
Postoperative analgesia:	II; PO medications
Acceptable techniques:	Local, spinal, epidural, GA

Comments: The anesthetic choice will depend on the surgeon's past experience, the size of the hernia, the patient's coexisting diseases, and your own desires.

Patients under local or regional can cough or strain on command to help demonstrate the defect, which is good. They are also less likely to cough or strain at the end of the case, which is even better. A solid T-6 level is necessary to block all stimuli from traction on the spermatic cord and lower peritoneum. Local anesthesia needs to be administered generously.

Patients under general anesthesia must be awakened and extubated smoothly to avoid stressing the surgeon's repair prematurely.

Traction on the viscera can cause typical vagal responses: bradycardia, hypotension, nausea, and vomiting.

The patient with a segment of bowel strangulated in the hernia may require emergency laparotomy and a bowel resection. These folks will be quite sick.

Hernia repairs can now be done laparoscopically, using a big sheet of Marlex stapled over the defect from the inside. The procedure tends to take a little longer to do, but the patient recovers much faster. And it's fun to watch. The usual laparoscopy concerns apply.

Ventral Hernia

Description: The surgeon opens the skin over the obvious bulging defect, frees up the fascial edges, and closes. Large defects with indistinct edges may require a sheet of Marlex mesh to secure things.

Position:	Supine
Estimated time:	30 minutes plus
Estimated blood loss:	Minimal
Need for muscle relaxation:	Required for closing fascia
Indicated monitors:	Standard
Postoperative analgesia:	II; PO medications
Acceptable techniques:	Spinal (T-4 level), GETA, local

Comments: Look at the patient's belly yourself before starting the case. This will give you some idea of how big the defect is and what sort of anesthetic will be required. Ask the surgeons whether they plan to use mesh (which takes longer) and if they anticipate a difficult dissection.

Small hernias (not extending to the peritoneum) can be done under local anesthesia. Even if the peritoneum is violated, sometimes you can get by spraying the exposed viscera with 1% lidocaine.

Epidural anesthesia will usually be too slow to provide an adequate block for this operation and may fail to provide adequate abdominal wall relaxation. A solid T-4 spinal will be much more comfortable for all concerned.

Coughing, bucking, and straining with emergence and extubation will prematurely test the surgical repair. If it falls apart you will find your popularity in sudden decline.

Peritoneal Dialysis Catheter Placement

Description: The surgeon makes a small incision above the umbilicus, reaches into the peritoneum, pulls up a segment of omentum, wraps it around the catheter, and stuffs the whole thing back into the belly.

Position:	Supine
Estimated time:	60 minutes
Estimated blood loss:	Minimal
Need for muscle relaxation:	Not necessary
Indicated monitors:	Standard
Postoperative analgesia:	II; PO medications
Acceptable techniques:	Local, GETA, spinal, epidural (T-3 level)

Comments: These patients are sick! (Why else would they need a dialysis catheter?) It's important to know why they are in renal failure and what other problems they might have. Take a good look at the labs to see what's out of whack.

Local anesthesia is not as great an approach as one might think, because of the omental wrap for the catheter. We've done it, but we had to spray lidocaine on the exposed omentum and viscera, and limp along on a lot of sedation. Check the patient's coagulation status before starting a regional anesthetic, though, since platelet dysfunction is common in this population.

This procedure is not over until the surgeon has run in a couple of liters of dialysate and run them back out again. It's amazing how often the damn thing doesn't work the first time.

Venous Access Catheter Placement

Description: The surgeons percutaneously stick the subclavian vein, thread in a catheter, then tunnel it back under the skin of the chest wall, so it can remain for weeks or months of future use. Catheter brand names include Groshong, Mediport, and Broviac.

Position:	Supine, Trendelenburg
Estimated time:	60 minutes
Estimated blood loss:	Minimal
Need for muscle relaxation:	Not needed
Indicated monitors:	Standard
Postoperative analgesia:	II; PO medications
Acceptable techniques:	Local, MAC, GA

Comments: The patients for this procedure are usually sick, or about to be. Healthy patients will have their catheters put in by the surgeons under local anesthesia; it's only the sick ones that will come to you. Neonates and infants are one such group. End-stage cancer and HIV patients are another.

MAC is usually sufficient and often safer than any other approach. Many of these patients have HIV or cancer, so check their medical histories carefully.

Wear your lead underwear! Many surgeons prefer to do this procedure under fluoroscopy.

Although general anesthesia by mask will usually work OK, your access to the airway will be somewhat limited by the surgeons. You may want to intubate the especially difficult patients.

Remember the possibility of pneumothorax, and make sure someone (meaning you) checks the postoperative chest x-ray.

Laceration of a great vessel, thoracic duct, or atrium will lead rapidly to exsanguination, pericardial tamponade, heroic opening of the chest, and (potentially) death.

Appendectomy

Description: The surgeons make a small incision just above the right groin, cut down into the peritoneum, fish out the appendix, ligate its mesentary, cut it off, cauterize and close the stump, and suture up.

Position:	Supine
Estimated time:	60 minutes
Estimated blood loss:	Minimal
Need for muscle relaxation:	Required for surgical exposure
Indicated monitors:	Standard
Postoperative analgesia:	III; IM or IV injections
Acceptable techniques:	GETA, spinal (T-2 level)

Comments: Usually an emergency case done outside of regular hours. The patient should always be thought to have a full stomach. Even if the patient hasn't eaten, the disease process causes an ileus.

Patients are often in significant pain preoperatively and may be hard to titrate to a good level intraoperatively. It's very easy to give too much narcotic to these patients.

Infiltration of the wound with local anesthetic as the surgeons are closing will significantly reduce postoperative pain and may make emergence a whole lot smoother.

Spinal anesthesia can be done but is usually not pretty. Peritoneal and visceral stimulation are hard to blunt without a high level, although a little ketamine sedation can be a big help.

Occasionally the surgeons are wrong about the diagnosis, and the procedure mutates into something longer and uglier (like an ovarian cancer operation, for instance).

We have recently noted a trend toward laparoscopic appendectomy, the argument being that the morbidity is lower if the surgeon is wrong about the diagnosis. This is good for the patient but bad for you, since the procedure will take about three times longer. See the discussion of laparoscopy in Chapter 1 if your surgeon is part of this brave new world.

Diagnostic Laparoscopy/Laparoscopic Appendectomy

Description: The surgeons make a small incision at the umbilicus, inflate the abdomen with carbon dioxide, stick a scope in, and look around. Additional entry ports can be made via stab incisions anywhere in the belly to allow access for retractors, snippers, cauterizers, staplers, and similar hardware. The appendix, once detached, is usually removed through the incision at the umbilicus.

Position:	Supine
Estimated time:	60 minutes
Estimated blood loss:	Minimal
Need for muscle relaxation:	Helpful
Indicated monitors:	Standard, Foley
Postoperative analgesia:	II; PO medications
Acceptable techniques:	GETA

Comments: This procedure, although longer than an open appendectomy, is less painful for the patient. Sometimes, of course, laparoscopy merely confirms the need for an immediate open appendectomy (as when the appendix is ruptured or stuck down); in this case, the patient loses. Other times, though, the laparoscopy reveals a ruptured ovarian cyst, gastroenteritis, or some other benign (nonsurgical) condition, and no further operating occurs; in this case the patient wins.

All of the usual laparoscopy concerns apply (see Chapter 1).

Most of these patients will be emergency cases, and anyone with a surgical abdomen should be considered to have a full stomach.

Laparoscopic appendectomy causes very little postoperative pain. Remember this when preparing for emergence. The case also has a tendency to end abruptly, leaving you holding the MAC, as it were. Plan accordingly.

Laparoscopic Cholecystectomy

Description: The surgeon makes a small incision at the umbilicus, inflates the peritoneum with carbon dioxide, and then inserts a fiberoptic scope and a camera. Further stab incisions are used for liver retractors and operating instruments. The cholecystic duct and artery are identified and clipped (sometimes with a pause to shoot some contrast medium into the biliary tree and take an x-ray, looking for stones), and then the gallbladder is dissected off the liver bed with a cauterizing tool. The specimen is removed through the umbilical incision and the belly is rinsed out, deflated, and closed.

Position:	Supine, steep reverse Trendelenburg
Estimated time:	90 minutes
Estimated blood loss:	Minimal
Need for muscle relaxation:	Helpful
Indicated monitors:	Standard, Foley
Postoperative analgesia:	II; IM injections or PO medications
Acceptable techniques:	GETA

Comments: The usual laparoscopic concerns apply (see Chapter 1). Unlike open cholecystectomies, laparoscopic procedures cause only modest amounts of pain.

An orogastric tube should be placed after induction to decompress the stomach and make it a smaller target for stray trocars.

This operation gets harder in patients who've had previous surgery and have adhesions as a result. Some small percentage (depending on the surgeon's experience) will wind up as open procedures, especially if the liver or gut is lacerated or the cholangiogram is positive for stones in the common duct.

If the patient has an ileus from an active gallbladder infection, or if the patient is overweight, a rapid-sequence intubation may be called for.

The question of avoiding narcotics because of their potential for causing biliary spasm (and mimicking common duct stones on the cholangiogram) is still somewhat open. Talk with the surgeon if you think it's going to be a problem intraop. Postop, there will be no problem.

The blood pressure may disappear when the patient's circulating blood volume pools in his or her feet with reverse Trendelenburg positioning.

Open Cholecystectomy

Description: Through a right subdiaphragmatic incision the surgeon exposes the gallbladder, ligates its artery and duct, and rips the sucker out. The presence of stones in the common bile duct (determined by palpation or cholangiogram) necessitates a more complicated exploration of the duct, all the way down to the duodenum, to make sure that no stones are left behind.

Position:	Supine
Estimated time:	2 hours
Estimated blood loss:	100 ml; type and cross-match 2 units
Need for muscle relaxation:	Required
Indicated monitors:	Standard
Postoperative analgesia:	III; patient-controlled analgesia or epidural
Acceptable techniques:	GETA, combined

Comments: This operation is very painful. The subdiaphragmatic incision violates a number of muscle layers that are strained by respiration. These patients are at high risk for postoperative atelectasis and pneumonia because of splinting on the operative side.

This operation is occasionally done on an emergency basis, during an active attack of cholecystitis. These patients should be thought to have full stomachs and should be well hydrated IV before their anesthetic. Anorexia, vomiting, and third-space losses around the gallbladder can all conspire to make the patient dehydrated.

In the very high-risk patient, a percutaneous cholecystostomy can be done under local anesthesia, but this approach is not recommended; the procedure is painful enough that your local anesthetic often becomes a general anesthetic despite the patient's condition.

Intraop narcotics may be contraindicated if the surgeon is concerned about the potential for biliary spasm. This is where regional anesthetic techniques for pain management (such as an epidural or rib blocks) become very helpful. Postop narcotics are fine.

Mastectomy/Axillary Node Dissection

Description: The skin and soft tissue of the breast is dissected off the chest wall, towards the axilla. The specimen is extended to include as many lymph nodes as can be found. The degree of malignancy of the tumor determines whether the muscles of the chest wall are taken as well.

Position:	Supine
Estimated time:	150 minutes
Estimated blood loss:	300 ml; type and cross-match 2 units
Need for muscle relaxation:	Not needed—may be contraindicated
Indicated monitors:	Standard
Postoperative analgesia:	III; PCA
Acceptable techniques:	GETA

Comments: This is almost always a cancer operation, and the usual concerns for cancer surgery apply (see Chapter 1). Postoperative pain can be very subjective.

Occasionally this procedure is followed by immediate reconstruction of the breast, sometimes with a saline implant. This adds a lot of time to the procedure but not much blood loss.

The surgeon may prefer that you don't use any muscle relaxation, so that he or she can see how close the dissection is coming to the long thoracic (or any other) nerve in the axilla.

The ipsilateral arm is typically prepped and part of the surgery, so your IV and all monitors must be placed on the other side.

Bleeding can be brisk for short portions of the dissection but is usually easily controlled.

Thyroid Lobectomy

Description: The surgeon makes a transverse ("throat slit") incision in the neck and exposes the thyroid on the side of interest. A slow dissection (the thyroid is extremely vascular, and the surgeon may be trying to leave the parathyroids behind) eventually frees up one-half the organ, which is removed. Closure is rapid.

Position:	Supine, shoulder bump with head back, neck extended, arms tucked at the sides, bed in semi-Fowler's position
Estimated time:	3 hours
Estimated blood loss:	200 ml; type and screen
Need for muscle relaxation:	May be contraindicated
Indicated monitors:	Standard
Postoperative analgesia:	II; PO medications
Acceptable techniques:	GETA only; no easy way to block

Comments: The dissection of the thyroid can be quite tedious and may present challenges for the anesthetist. Surgical stimulation is minimal, except when the surgeon suddenly stimulates the trachea. Since the patient is usually not paralyzed (so the surgeon will know when a nerve is whacked), this invariably causes the patient to cough or buck, and generates sarcastic remarks such as "You can put the patient to sleep now, we've started," and "It's OK, Mrs. Smith, you're doing fine." We suggest you either keep the patient a little deeper than the vital signs might indicate or develop a solid repertoire of snappy rejoinders.

On the other hand, the operation ends very quickly and the postoperative pain is minimal, meaning that wake-ups can be slow and difficult if the patient is on the deep side. Consider using agents that are easy to get rid of, like propofol or desflurane.

Exciting intraoperative events include the sudden development of thyroid storm (rare) and that stimulating wait for the frozen section report to come back from pathology (all too common).

Postoperative excitement can be generated by pneumothorax, hypocalcemic crisis, vocal cord paresis (unusual with unilateral surgery), or hematoma. A little bleeding in the thyroid bed will lead to early compression of the lymphatic and venous drainage from the trachea, leading to impressive and potentially lethal upper airway edema. The surgeon will have a low threshold for returning the patient to the OR to re-explore the neck, and you should have a very low threshold for reintubating if things don't look right.

Total Thyroidectomy/ Parathyroidectomy

Description: Through a transverse neck incision, the surgeons mobilize the thyroid (usually a tedious process) and remove it. In the case of thyroid surgery, they will try and identify the parathyroids and leave them in place.

Position:	Supine, reverse Trendelenburg, arms tucked, shoulders bumped up, head back
Estimated time:	4 hours
Estimated blood loss:	200 ml; type and cross-match 2 units
Need for muscle relaxation:	May be contraindicated
Indicated monitors:	Standard
Postoperative analgesia:	II; surprisingly little postoperative pain
Acceptable techniques:	GETA

Comments: As with thyroid lobectomies (see previous procedure), one must be concerned with keeping the anesthetic at an effective level without muscle relaxants. Additional concerns include thyroid storm, pneumothorax, hematoma, slow dissection, and protracted waiting for the pathology report.

Removal of all four parathyroids will lead to hypocalcemia, occurring over 4–6 hours and typically manifested by respiratory weakness and then stridor in the PACU. This is one of the great zebras of anesthesia and well worth remembering anytime you see tissue removed from the neck.

With a bilateral operation you should be concerned with injury to the recurrent laryngeal nerves and bilateral vocal cord paresis. The surgeon may want you to assess vocal cord function postoperatively, which can be difficult to do. One approach is to let the patient wake up all the way, extubate, topicalize, and go in for a look with the bronchoscope. This is somewhat cumbersome. Another approach is to extubate deep (real deep) on a volatile anesthetic, with the patient breathing sponta-neously, and then look at the cords via direct laryn-goscopy. If you are smart enough to have used desflurane as your agent, you can then wake the patient right up and head for the golf course. If you used isoflurane, it may take a little longer.

Most major neck surgery patients will make extended stays in the PACU for observation. Then when they do get stridorous (typically from their hematoma), you can hustle them right back into the OR and tackle their air-way under the best possible circumstances.

Vagotomy/Pyloroplasty

Description: Through a midline upper abdominal incision, the surgeon finds the pylorus and opens it longitudinally. It is then closed horizontally, effectively making it several times wider. This allows acid from the stomach to drain freely into the duodenum, instead of pooling and causing ulcers. The "vagotomy" part means that the surgeon will scrape all the nerves possible off the gastric body, reducing its innervation and (hopefully) its desire to produce acid.

Position:	Supine
Estimated time:	2 hours
Estimated blood loss:	400 ml; type and cross-match 2 units
Need for muscle relaxation:	Essential for surgical exposure
Indicated monitors:	Standard, Foley, A-line for unstable patients
Postoperative analgesia:	III; PCA or epidural
Acceptable techniques:	GETA; combined

Comments: This operation is most commonly done on an emergency basis, in a patient with an intractable gastric ulcer. Laser coagulators, selective vasopressin injections (Pitressin), and six-port operating endoscopes have given the gastroenterologists a lot more tools to work with before calling the surgeons, so this operation is not nearly as common as it used to be. On the other hand, the patients we do see have already had the old college try, and may be the worse for it. Expect them to be severely volume depleted, anemic, and potentially very unstable.

Needless to say, these patients should be treated as full stomachs. In addition, think for a moment about why they got the ulcer in the first place. Alcoholism is a common reason and may complicate your anesthetic.

Have blood and abundant IV access available. Use a blood and airway warmer. Keep the patient covered and the room warm.

Be wary of severe hypotension from using an epidural in a hypovolemic patient.

Keep an eye on what the surgeons are doing. The upper abdomen is expensive real estate, and a blunder into the liver or celiac plexus may be lethal.

Splenectomy

Description: Through either a midline or left lateral incision, the surgeon dissects the spleen out of its bed, ligates the splenic artery, ties the splenic vein(s), and removes the specimen. This surgery may be done for trauma, idiopathic thrombocytopenic purpura, lymphoma, various cancers, or because the splenic artery has been sacrificed in some other cause (such as a Whipple or Billroth procedure).

Position:	Supine, left side bumped up, or right lateral decubitus
Estimated time:	3 hours
Estimated blood loss:	500 ml; type and cross-match 2 units
Need for muscle relaxation:	Required
Indicated monitors:	Standard, Foley; consider A-line
Postoperative analgesia:	IV; may be extremely painful
Acceptable techniques:	GETA, combined

Comments: Normal spleens are relatively easy to remove surgically but are typically found in trauma patients who may be hypovolemic and unstable. Abnormal spleens may be small and shrunken (easy) or very large (difficult).

Rapid bleeding can occur but is usually easy to control. Of course, if the bleeding starts before the surgery does (as in a trauma patient), you may have to transfuse the patient before the incision is even made. Be prepared with lots of IV access, fluid and airway heaters, and a warm room.

Rarely, the surgical approach will wander across the diaphragm. Be aware of the potential for a pneumothorax postoperatively, and don't be surprised if the surgeon suddenly asks for a chest tube.

This scarcely matters to the anesthetist, but splenectomy patients all need preoperative vaccination against encapsulated bacteria.

The patient with ITP may present with a very low platelet count, which will prevent you from doing a regional anesthetic. You will want to check with the hematologist beforehand to satisfy yourself that everything possible has been done to prepare the patient medically (steroids, gamma globulin), and you should talk to the blood bank about having platelets ready for transfusion.

Bowel Resection

Description: Through a midline incision the surgeons open the peritoneum, free the gut from whatever adhesions may be holding it down, remove the section they want as specimen, reattach the ends, and close. In an emergency case (unprepped bowel) the surgeon may create a colostomy rather than primarily reconnecting the bowel.

Position:	Supine
Estimated time:	3 hours
Estimated blood loss:	300 ml; type and cross-match 2 units
Need for muscle relaxation:	Required
Indicated monitors:	Standard, Foley; consider A-line
Postoperative analgesia:	III; PCA, intrathecal narcotics, or epidural infusion
Acceptable techniques:	GETA, GETA combined with epidural/intrathecal

Comments: This is a common cancer surgery (see Chapter 1). Colon cancer commonly metastasizes to the lungs and liver, so you will want to carefully check the chest x-ray report and liver function tests before starting.

Most of these patients will have received a generous bowel prep preoperatively. Manufacturers' claims notwithstanding, this means that they will be significantly dehydrated when you meet them.

Although bleeding is not usually a big problem, third-space fluid and heat losses can be substantial. Use your warmers.

Nitrous oxide may be contraindicated if there is an element of bowel obstruction, or if the surgeon is having a hard time closing. Contrary to what you may have heard, nitrous will usually be OK in the bowel-prepped patient with a good epidural.

Epidural blockade and sympathectomy may constrict the bowel, potentially making it harder to suture. This effect can be reversed with IV anticholinergic drugs (atropine or glycopyrrolate).

Colostomy Takedown

Description: Sounds like a professional wrestling move, doesn't it? In fact this operation simply consists of the surgeon reconnecting two previously separated pieces of bowel, usually after enough time has passed to allow healing of the primary disease. The same midline incision is used, and, after some tedious dissection, the two free ends are found, shortened somewhat ("freshened"), and reconnected. Closure includes closure of the colostomy hole.

Position:	Supine
Estimated time:	3 hours
Estimated blood loss:	300 ml; type and cross-match 2 units
Need for muscle relaxation:	Required for surgical exposure
Indicated monitors:	Standard, Foley, A-line
Postoperative analgesia:	III
Acceptable techniques:	GETA, combined

Comments: This patient will surely have had a generous bowel prep preoperatively, which will make them hypovolemic and sensitive to anesthetic agents.

Adhesions are likely on the second trip into a given patient's belly, so this procedure can become longer than advertised. Temperature and third-space fluid loss are big concerns.

The good news is that the heat is usually off on the cancer watch. If the original cancer hadn't been cured, you probably wouldn't be doing this procedure.

As with bowel resections, the use of an epidural anesthetic can shrink the gut and make the reanastomosis harder for the surgeon. IV atropine or glycopyrrolate will reverse this process, however.

Nitrous oxide will distend the gut (in the absence of an epidural) and may make closure difficult. We usually use it until we either see the gut expanding or hear the surgeon complain, at which point we turn it off. Distension due to nitrous oxide will reverse over 15–30 minutes.

Diaphragmatic Hernia Repair (Adult)

Description: The surgeon opens the belly and dissects north, attempting to pull all the abdominal contents back into the abdomen, define the defect in the diaphragm, and close it. Sometimes Marlex mesh is used to cover up a big hole.

Position:	Supine or lateral decubitus
Estimated time:	3 hours
Estimated blood loss:	300 ml; type and cross-match 2 units
Need for muscle relaxation:	Required
Indicated monitors:	Standard, Foley, A-line
Postoperative analgesia:	IV
Acceptable techniques:	GETA, combined

Comments: Plan on a chest tube postoperatively.

No nitrous oxide please; closing the belly may be hard as it is.

Ventilating by hand, while watching what the surgeon is doing, can make some parts of the dissection much faster.

As with any belly case, temperature and third-space fluid losses will be very important concerns.

The liver, spleen, stomach, or lung can all get in the way of the procedure and be inadvertently damaged. Make sure you have enough IV access to deal with any sudden crisis.

No matter what surgical approach is used, this incision will hurt like hell afterwards. Be prepared to use your big guns for postop analgesia.

Small Bowel Obstruction

Description: This procedure typically is done on an emergency basis. The surgical goal is to open the belly, figure out what's obstructing the bowel, and fix it. This may mean taking down a few adhesions and straightening out a volvulus; it may mean correcting a ventral or inguinal hernia; or it may mean creating a diverting ileostomy around a huge tumor or infectious mass.

Position:	Supine
Estimated time:	2 hours plus
Estimated blood loss:	300 ml plus; type and crossmatch 2 units
Need for muscle relaxation:	Required for surgical exposure
Indicated monitors:	Standard, Foley, low threshold for A-line, central line
Postoperative analgesia:	III
Acceptable techniques:	GETA, rarely combined

Comments: All patients have full stomachs, with a high risk for aspiration. Metoclopramide is contraindicated as a prophylactic agent.

Expect the patient to be severely dehydrated secondary to vomiting and to third-space fluid loss into the obstructed gut. Be generous with fluids preoperatively, be gentle when inducing anesthesia, and use caution with your epidural sympathectomy.

Check the electrolytes preoperatively. Preoperative fluid loss into the gut wall can really screw things up.

The operation can take anywhere from a few minutes to all day. Be prepared to keep the patient warm and well hydrated, and don't be afraid to add monitors or IV access as you go along.

No nitrous!

Nissen Fundoplication: Open or Laparoscopic

Description: The goal of the surgeon is to wrap the gastric fundus around the abdominal esophagus and secure it there, tightening the lower esophageal sphincter and preventing reflux.

Position:	Supine
Estimated time:	4 hours
Estimated blood loss:	500 ml
Need for muscle relaxation:	Required
Indicated monitors:	Standard, Foley, A-line
Postoperative analgesia:	IV
Acceptable techniques:	GETA, combined

Comments: Treat the patient as if he or she has a full stomach. Provide aspiration prophylaxis preoperatively and plan on a rapid-sequence induction.

Intraoperatively the surgeons will ask you to pass a bougie esophageal dilator into the stomach (to give them a stent to tighten around). This is not usually hard, if you remember to lubricate the bougie well. Be careful when removing the bougie, however; it's embarrassing to simultaneously extubate the patient.

As with any major upper abdominal surgery, the dissection can be tedious and fraught with potential pitfalls. You must keep the patient warm and well hydrated in the face of significant third-space losses.

Inadvertent transgression of the diaphragm can occur. Be wary of a pneumothorax!

This operation is now being done laparoscopically. All of the usual laparoscopic considerations apply (see Chapter 1). The position is slightly different; the surgeon stands between the patient's legs, looking at a TV screen at the head of the bed, and a little reverse Trendelenburg is usually applied. Blood, fluid, and heat losses are minimal, no A-line is needed, and postoperative pain is only a II.

Abdominal Perineal Resection (APR)

Description: This operation is performed for rectal or low sigmoid cancers, or occasionally for severe ulcerative colitis or Crohn's disease. The sigmoid colon is dissected free from within the belly, and the rectum is dissected from the perineal side. When the dissections meet, the specimen is removed. Closure involves either a colostomy or an immediate ileo-anal pull-through.

Position:	Lithotomy
Estimated time:	5 hours
Estimated blood loss:	700 ml; type and cross-match 4 units
Need for muscle relaxation:	Required for surgical exposure
Indicated monitors:	Standard, Foley, A-line, CVP/PA line
Postoperative analgesia:	III
Acceptable techniques:	GETA, combined

Comments: All these patients will be facing a major loss of function; see the section on cancer surgery in Chapter 1 for the appropriate considerations.

The preoperative bowel prep inflicted on the patient by the surgeon will make your induction very exciting if you don't provide adequate hydration first.

This will be a long case with significant third-space heat and fluid loss. Blood loss is rarely brisk but can add up to a significant amount by the end of the day.

Epidural blockade of the sympathetic nerves will cause the gut to contract, potentially making the surgeon's job harder. If he or she complains, try giving some IV atropine to reverse the effect.

Nitrous oxide may need to be turned off toward the end of the case, if the gut is swollen enough to make closure difficult.

Billroth Gastrectomy

Description: Through a midline incision the surgeon frees up the stomach and then removes the lower two-thirds of it. The duodenal stump is oversewn, and the remaining portion of the stomach is connected to a Roux-en-Y piece of jejunum. This operation may be done for intractable ulcer disease or for gastric carcinoma.

Position:	Supine
Estimated time:	5 hours
Estimated blood loss:	1,000 ml; type and cross-match 4 units
Need for muscle relaxation:	Required
Indicated monitors:	Standard, Foley, A-line, CVP/PA line
Postoperative analgesia:	IV
Acceptable techniques:	GETA, combined

Comments: Patients who present for a Billroth procedure will usually be quite sick. Either they will be bleeding profusely and hemodynamically unstable, or they will have a carcinoma and be depressed, malnourished, and anemic.

All these patients should be treated as if they have full stomachs.

Elective patients will have had a thorough bowel prepping, meaning that they will be dehydrated and sensitive to anesthetics.

This is a big operation! The patient will get cold very quickly and will probably soak up oceans of crystalloid. Be prepared to manage these problems from the very beginning of the case.

This is the high-rent district of the abdomen. Surgical misadventure can lead into the liver, spleen, pancreas, or even across the diaphragm. Be prepared to handle crises if they arise.

Prepare the patient for a long, hard postoperative recovery. Don't plan on extubating unless things go perfectly, and be prepared to use your best analgesic plan postop.

Pancreas Resection (Whipple)

Description: Through a midline abdominal incision, the surgeon dissects down to the retroperitoneum and removes the pancreas and duodenum as a block. The stomach is connected to one Roux-en-Y piece of jejunum, and the bile duct to another. The tail of the pancreas may go or stay, depending on the disease process.

Position:	Supine
Estimated time:	6 hours plus
Estimated blood loss:	1,500 ml plus; type and crossmatch 6 units
Need for muscle relaxation:	Required
Indicated monitors:	Standard, Foley, A-line, PA line
Postoperative analgesia:	IV
Acceptable techniques:	GETA, combined

Comments: This operation is usually performed for cancer (see Chapter 1) and can end abruptly if metastatic disease is found in the liver or elsewhere in the belly. Rarely, this surgery is performed for chronic pancreatitis. In either case the patient is apt to be malnourished and anemic preoperatively.

Yes, these patients are bowel prepped. They will start the day already somewhat dehydrated.

This is one of the hardest dissections of all for the general surgeon. Sometimes when they get in around the porta hepatis, the bleeding just doesn't stop. Be prepared with lots of IV access, and give coagulation factors and platelets early if it looks like things aren't going well.

If you are using an epidural, be careful with the sympathectomy. Don't do anything that will embarrass you later in the case.

Warmth and adequate hydration will be big concerns from the very start.

If the blood pressure falls suddenly, check on what the surgeons are doing. Deliberate or inadvertent compression of the inferior vena cava may abruptly drop the preload to the heart and erase the blood pressure in a matter of a few beats.

Nitrous oxide may be problematic late in the case. Turn it off if you have to.

These patients deserve aggressive postoperative pain relief. Continuous epidural analgesia may be enormously beneficial, if the patient is hemodynamically stable.

Liver Resection

Description: The belly is opened, the offending section of the liver is identified, and the bleeding commences. Various devices including lasers and ultrasonic dissectors may be used in an attempt to control blood loss, but they are not always as effective as you hope they might be.

Position:	Supine
Estimated time:	6 hours
Estimated blood loss:	2,000 ml plus; type and crossmatch 6 units; consider fresh-frozen plasma (FFP) and platelets
Need for muscle relaxation:	Required
Indicated monitors:	Standard, Foley, A-line, PA line, frequent labs
Postoperative analgesia:	IV
Acceptable techniques:	GETA

Comments: These patients may have cancer or other systemic disease (such as alcoholism). Check the lab studies carefully before starting the case for evidence of malnutrition or preexisting coagulopathies.

Bleeding is the big issue with liver surgery. The liver just does not take sutures well, and the nearby large vessels can be impossible to repair if damaged. You should plan to have an abundance of vascular access and your best possible system for warming and administering large volumes of fluid.

Make the decision to use FFP and/or platelets early if it looks like there's a lot of bleeding. Coagulopathy is common and very hard to recover from.

Keep the patient warm from the beginning.

Don't count on extubating postoperatively unless everything has gone perfectly. An epidural is a good idea for postoperative pain management but should be dosed with extreme care in the OR. A little sympathectomy can drastically worsen things for you and the patient if excessive bleeding occurs.

Adrenalectomy

Description: The retroperitoneum is accessed via the lower ribs, which are either spread out of the way or removed. The vascular connections of the adrenal are carefully identified and ligated, and the gland is removed.

Position:	Lateral decubitus, as for a kidney
Estimated time:	4 hours
Estimated blood loss:	500 ml; type and cross-match 4 units
Need for muscle relaxation:	Required
Indicated monitors:	Standard, Foley, A-line, CVP or PA for drug infusion
Postoperative analgesia:	IV
Acceptable techniques:	GETA, combined

Comments: This operation may be done for a variety of adrenal tumors but most especially a pheochromocytoma. The patient will generally be healthy otherwise, although some will have other endocrine tumors that affect your anesthetic plans. Most important for you in your preoperative assessment will be figuring out what factors the patient's tumor is secreting and what is going to happen when it is removed.

Pheochromocytomas secrete catecholamines, including epinephrine, norepinephrine, and dopamine. The patient will present initially with tachycardia and impressive intermittent hypertension. The exact factors released can be determined by analyzing the patient's urine, which you should check on preoperatively. The patient who has had an elevated catecholamine level for a long time will be chronically volume depleted and may have a cardiomyopathy and abnormal autoregulatory ranges for the brain and kidneys.

Preoperatively, it is imperative to normalize the patient's hemodynamics. This process usually begins with PO alpha-antagonists, like phenoxybenzamine, titrated to give the patient a mild case of orthostatic hypotension, which is treated with volume expansion.

Once the blood pressure is under control, beta blockers are added to bring the heart rate down. Not only will hemodynamic normalization make your anesthetic smoother in the face of surgical stressors and direct manipulation of the tumor, but it may also make the patient more stable postoperatively. Sudden removal of a secreting tumor can leave the patient with a misadjusted "set point" and force you to infuse catecholamines postoperatively until the patient can readjust. It's better to get the patient normalized preoperatively so that they don't miss the tumor when it's gone.

An epidural anesthetic, with a near-total sympathectomy, is one way to minimize hemodynamic perturbations during the case. IV nitroprusside is another. No matter what method is chosen and how well the patient is prepared preoperatively, you can expect a real roller coaster ride with the patient's blood pressure. If it's any consolation, the patient has probably been yo-yoing up and down on their own for months previously.

Hormonal considerations aside, an adrenalectomy is still a major operation. The patient must be kept warm and well hydrated, and transfusion may be required if the resection becomes excessively gory.

A good epidural analgesic may make it possible to extubate the patient at the conclusion of the procedure, but don't push your luck. If you've given a lot of fluid, if the patient has been especially unstable, or if the patient's coexisting diseases are significant enough, you may just want to keep the patient intubated and anesthetized all the way to the ICU.

Patients undergoing bilateral adrenalectomy will require stress steroid coverage.

Ear, Nose, and Throat Surgery

Non-neurologic surgery above the clavicles spans a wide range of cases, from 15-minute tonsillectomies to 20-hour radical neck resections; a wide range of patients, from 3-year-olds for myringotomies to 80-year-olds for acoustic neuroma resections; and a wide range of seriousness, from ear operations to vocal cord biopsies. ENT cases can be incredibly demanding and stimulating, such as a jet ventilation IV anesthetic for an upper airway laser case. They can also be mind-numbingly dull, such as an 8-hour ossicular reconstruction in a healthy 24-year-old.

The big anesthetic concern in ENT surgery is who is responsible for the airway and when. In many of these procedures this duty must be shared, and it is important for you and the surgeon to communicate. A good ENT surgeon can teach you a lot about the anatomy of the upper airway and can be a valuable resource when things get sticky in the OR or PACU. A bad ENT surgeon, on the other hand, can set you up for disasters beyond your imagining. When making your plans for airway management in an ENT case, there are two things you must always do: (1) talk with the surgeon to make sure you are on the same page, (2) and have a back-up plan in case the first one doesn't work out. As always, make sure the tube is secured when you're not looking at it, and make sure you have all the equipment you might need in an emergency.

Another feature of the ENT service is that a large part of their business is same-day surgery for tonsils, ears, and sinuses. You will have to learn how to adjust your anesthetics to facilitate the rapid turnover expected on a busy ENT day. Concentrate on having your patients wake up crisply, without excessive pain or nausea.

You will also have to learn how to assess patients in the PACU. Is that stridor just a little upper airway edema that'll go down with time, or are you already too late with the tracheostomy? Just how much blood has little Johnny swallowed? And how do people get that bluish color anyway? ENT patients deserve closer watching than many, because they can bleed in occult ways and because their airways can get worse even after being wide awake for extubation. They may also get large doses of local anesthetics, which can produce toxic reactions from overdose or intravascular injection.

Several of the cases that follow are also reproduced in the pediatric surgery chapter (Chapter 11).

Bilateral Myringotomy and Tubes (Ear Tubes) (BMTT)

Description: This staple of the ENT service is done through an operating microscope. A small incision is made in the eardrum and a little grommet is inserted to keep the hole open. Steroid eardrops are drizzled in to reduce swelling, the external ear is packed with cotton, and you're finished.

Position:	Supine
Estimated time:	15 minutes
Estimated blood loss:	Minimal
Need for muscle relaxation:	None
Indicated monitors:	Standard
Postoperative analgesia:	II; PO medications
Acceptable techniques:	GA

Comments: Typically done under mask anesthesia, with the patient breathing spontaneously, and with the surgeon and anesthetist working together to stay out of each other's way.

In the routine pediatric case, you can skip the IV (although you should have everything necessary on hand). Have an IM dose of succinylcholine and atropine handy, though, just in case you run into trouble. These cases are usually so fast that you should plan on completing your anesthetic record in the PACU.

Because this operation is done in kids with chronic ear infections, you may have to accept a certain amount of sniffling and upper respiratory infection symptoms in your patient. Things that might make you cancel an elective hernia repair can be tolerated here, because the patient may never get any better. Usually you are able to maintain spontaneous ventilation and avoid an endotracheal tube. Still, be prepared for laryngospasm and other airway problems.

Tonsillectomy/Adenoidectomy

Description: Operating through the mouth, the surgeon curettes the tonsillar and/or adenoidal tissue off the side of the pharynx, does something about the bleeding, and leaves.

Position:	Supine, bed turned away from the anesthetist
Estimated time:	45 minutes
Estimated blood loss:	50 ml; type and screen
Need for muscle relaxation:	Not necessary
Indicated monitors:	Standard
Postoperative analgesia:	II; PO medications, local injection by surgeon
Acceptable techniques:	GETA, local

Comments: Although previously performed mostly for tonsillitis, obstructive apnea is presently the leading reason for tonsillectomy/adenoidectomy. As with ear tubes, you may have to accept a certain amount of preoperative illness on the part of the patient, since he or she may have a continuous upper respiratory infection or tonsillitis until this operation is done.

The surgeon will typically use a special tonsillar gag to hold the mouth open and expose the pharynx. This gag holds your (oral) endotracheal tube in the midline of the tongue. Your circuit will typically approach from the patient's chest. Using a tube designed to make a sharp corner southward from the mouth (RAE or Flexibend) will help you avoid embarrassing tube kink incidents. Keep the circuit taped to the patient's chest, and pay special attention to the airway; there will be several episodes of disconnection and reconnection of your circuit while the surgeon is getting the gag positioned.

Blood in the airway is a wonderful stimulant for laryngospasm. Make sure the surgeon has suctioned the patient thoroughly before you attempt to extubate.

If the surgeon uses a throat pack to keep blood out of the stomach, make sure it gets removed at the end of the case, and document this fact on your anesthetic record. And don't forget to suction out the stomach anyway.

The surgeon may be planning to send the patient

home on the day of surgery, but this approach may not always be reasonable, especially in young children who presented with obstructive apnea. Think about this issue as you drop the child in the PACU.

Blood loss postoperatively can vanish invisibly into the stomach, leaving patients significantly hypovolemic (and with a full stomach) when you take them back to the OR to correct the bleeding. This oral boards favorite situation is best approached with an IV rapid-sequence induction, after initial hydration, using an agent like ketamine that won't embarrass you.

In children, try hard to place and secure the IV so that it has a reasonable chance of surviving intact and functioning through the wake-up and early postop period. It may save your neck if the patient needs to come back to the OR on an emergency basis.

In cooperative adults, this procedure can be done under local anesthesia alone. Just not on any of us.

Endoscopic Sinus Surgery (FESS)

Description: Using a rigid magnifying scope with a fiberoptic light source, the surgeons root around in the patient's nose. They can drain sinuses, excise unnecessary tissue (like polyps), and cauterize bleeding points. With luck, they stay out of the carotid artery, brain, and eyeball, all of which are nearby.

Position:	Semi-Fowler's (half sitting up)
Estimated time:	120 minutes
Estimated blood loss:	Minimal (may have ongoing occult loss)
Need for muscle relaxation:	Not needed
Indicated monitors:	Standard
Postoperative analgesia:	II; PO medications
Acceptable techniques:	GETA, MAC, local

Comments: Many surgeons do this operation predominantly under local, meaning that the only patients you will see will be old, sick, uncooperative, or all three.

Newer equipment, including good cameras and TV screens, has led to an indirect surgical technique. This allows the staff surgeon to supervise the resident's every move, which may make things faster or slower. It also means that you can watch the operation yourself, which does a lot to relieve the tedium.

With either anesthetic plan the surgeons will topicalize the nose to minimize bleeding. This will be done with lidocaine with epinephrine, cocaine, or phenylephrine, all of which can produce interesting hemodynamic side effects.

Your access to the airway will be limited once things get going, so if you have any doubts, intubate the patient up front. Secure the tube well once it goes in; you won't be seeing it again for a while.

Blood in the posterior pharynx can produce laryngospasm after extubation. Suction the patient well. Also be cognizant of the throat pack placed by the surgeons to alleviate this problem: You must make very sure that all of the throat packs that go in also come out. Document this on your record.

Uvulopalatopharyngoplasty (UPPP)

Description: To relieve sleep apnea or excessive snoring, the surgeons reach into the back of the mouth and resect any redundant tissue they can find, while tightening up the rest to keep the uvula suspended a little higher.

Position:	Supine
Estimated time:	120 minutes
Estimated blood loss:	200 ml; type and screen
Need for muscle relaxation:	Not necessary
Indicated monitors:	Standard
Postoperative analgesia:	II; PO medications
Acceptable techniques:	GETA

Comments: These patients can be very challenging to intubate, so a thorough airway exam is a good idea preop. Some surgeons will operate around an oral tube, like a tonsillectomy; others prefer a nasal intubation. It's usually a good idea to check with the surgeons before starting.

Aspiration prophylaxis is a good idea in many of these patients (the obese ones or those in whom you anticipate a slow intubation).

At the end of the procedure, you should help the surgeons count the throat packs as they take them out. Thorough suctioning is also a good idea to minimize the laryngospastic potential of blood in the airway.

Postoperatively these folks can have trouble with bleeding or with airway edema, either of which will ruin your day. Keep them sitting up, give them humidified oxygen to breathe, and get the ENT surgeon back to the bedside at the first sign of trouble.

Parotidectomy

Description: The surgeons will make an incision just in front of the ear and delicately remove the parotid gland from its comfortable embrace of the facial nerve. A pathology-proven malignancy may also lead to modified or radical neck dissection.

Position:	Supine, with head turned
Estimated time:	180 minutes
Estimated blood loss:	Minimal
Need for muscle relaxation:	May be contraindicated
Indicated monitors:	Standard
Postoperative analgesia:	II; PO medications
Acceptable techniques:	GETA

Comments: The use of neuromuscular blocking agents should be discussed with the surgeons ahead of time. They may prefer you to keep the patient unparalyzed so that they can see the lips twitch as they dissect around the facial nerve.

If you're not using paralysis to keep the patient still, be wary of overanesthetizing. This operation doesn't cause much pain, and waking up from a deep anesthetic will be slow.

The length of the case will be variable, depending on the degree of involvement of the tumor with the facial nerve.

You will have no access to the patient's head once the surgery begins. Tape the endotracheal tube like you mean it! (But don't get the tape in the surgeon's way, of course.)

Mastoidectomy/Tympanoplasty—Any Ear Case

Description: The surgeons pull the external ear forward and enter the middle and inner ear, using a drill to get there and a microscope to operate with once they arrive.

Position:	Supine, head turned to the side
Estimated time:	240 very long minutes
Estimated blood loss:	Minimal
Need for muscle relaxation:	Discuss with the surgeon
Indicated monitors:	Standard, Foley
Postoperative analgesia:	II; PO medications
Acceptable techniques:	GETA

Comments: Discuss the use of neuromuscular blocking agents with the surgeon before you start. In some ear cases, monitoring the function of the facial nerve is indicated, meaning that muscle relaxation must be avoided.

If you're not using muscle relaxants, plan on a deeper anesthetic. Having the patient move while under the microscope is somewhat embarrassing.

Check with the surgeons again at the end of the case. Depending on how the middle and inner ear are closed, it may be best to discontinue the use of nitrous oxide for the last hour or so of the case.

Bring a good book. It's going to be a long, slow day.

Acoustic Neuroma

Description: The ENT surgeon, sometimes assisted by a neurosurgeon, drills a hole through the mastoid to get to the neuroma, then resects as much of it as possible.

Position:	Supine, head away
Estimated time:	8 hours
Estimated blood loss:	200 ml; type and cross-match 2 units
Need for muscle relaxation:	Usually contraindicated
Indicated monitors:	Standard, Foley, A-line
Postoperative analgesia:	II, PO medications
Acceptable techniques:	GETA

Comments: Because of the plethora of nerves that can be tangled up in the tumor, muscle relaxation is contraindicated so that evoked potential and facial nerve monitoring can take place.

These are long cases, but the incision is small and blood, fluid, and heat losses are all usually modest. If the surgeons get into the carotid, though, all bets are off.

Inner ear disruption can cause nausea and vomiting postoperatively. Cranial nerve irritation can cause deafness, vertigo, and difficulty swallowing.

The airway will be difficult to access once the case gets started. Make sure the endotracheal tube is well secured.

Check out the section on posterior fossa surgery in the neurosurgery chapter (Chapter 13) for more information on this sort of procedure.

Depending on the nature of the tumor, the usual psychological considerations for cancer surgery may apply (see Chapter 1).

Upper Airway Surgery

Description: This category includes laser excision of pharyngeal masses, vocal cord biopsies, tongue resections, and a variety of similar transoral procedures.

Position:	Supine
Estimated time:	60 minutes
Estimated blood loss:	Minimal
Need for muscle relaxation:	May be helpful
Indicated monitors:	Standard
Postoperative analgesia:	II; oral medications
Acceptable techniques:	GETA

Comments: The most important feature of these cases is that you and the surgeon will be in a constant tug-of-war over the airway. The best way to avoid critical incidents is to work out a plan in advance, even if that means talking to the surgeon ahead of time. Good questions to ask are: Is the patient a hard intubation? Do you want a nasal tube? Will the patient remain intubated postop? Do we need the jet ventilator? Are you going to use a laser?

If a laser is involved in the vicinity of the vocal cords, consider jet ventilation through the operating laryngoscope and a total IV anesthetic. Check out the section on lasers in Chapter 1.

If you are planning to extubate postoperatively (and you usually are), think hard about airway edema before doing so. Suction thoroughly to avoid blood-induced laryngospasm. And make sure that all the throat packs and other hardware placed by the surgeons have been removed first.

Total Laryngectomy/Radical Neck Dissection

Description: Pretty much like it sounds. The surgeon opens the neck, takes out the tumor, takes out anything touching the tumor, takes out anything touching anything touching the tumor, and so forth. In the worst case, all that are left are vertebral bodies, carotid arteries, and a few nerves. Once everything is removed, the remaining large hole may require a muscle flap and skin graft to close.

Position:	Supine, often with the head turned
Estimated time:	12 hours, including reconstruction time
Estimated blood loss:	1,000 ml; type and cross-match 4 units
Need for muscle relaxation:	May be contraindicated
Indicated monitors:	Standard, Foley, A-Line; consider CVP/PA line
Postoperative analgesia:	III, PCA
Acceptable techniques:	GETA

Comments: Placing a central line that will not be in the surgeon's way can be difficult. Sometimes a subclavian is OK. Other times a long line from the arm or groin is needed.

The usual cancer surgery considerations apply (see Chapter 1). This will be a big, long case. Check out the sections on blood loss and temperature in Chapter 1. Fluid requirements may be increased due to the length of the procedure, the extent of the dissection, and the patient's poor nutritional status.

Surgical manipulation of the carotid body can produce sudden bradycardias. This is usually best prevented by surgical injection of 1% lidocaine into the vicinity of the carotid. The lidocaine should already be up on the surgical field so that it can be given expeditiously.

Open neck veins during the procedure can lead to venous air embolism, which is catastrophic. Aggressive surgical exploration can lead to tension pneumothorax, which is also catastrophic. Be prepared.

The airway may be compromised preoperatively by whatever disease process has lead to the surgery. Perform a careful exam up front and consider an awake fiberoptic intubation if things look ugly. Intraoperatively, the surgeons will often perform a tracheostomy, which makes things easy later on. If not, be very leery of extubating the patient. Airway edema from venous and lymphatic interruption and vocal cord paresis from surgical abuse can lead to rapid decompensation following extubation.

Gynecology

On the GYN service, all the patients are women, and many are nervous. Some are nervous because they have cancer or think they do; some are nervous because they are trying to get pregnant; and some are nervous because they're young and have never had surgery before.

For the most part, the patients will be healthy, with few problems other than whatever brings them to the OR. Thyroid disease is not uncommon, nor are chronic mild anemia or mild to moderate obesity. Most of the patients will be middle-aged or younger. The exceptions are the rare elderly oncology patients. Advanced ovarian carcinoma will make the patient as sick as anyone you'll ever meet, with ascitic fluid accumulating through the surgery almost faster than it can be sucked out.

Not surprisingly, good personal communication skills are essential to your survival on the GYN service. You must let the patient know that you are as concerned about her illness as she is, that you are going to take the best possible care of her, and that you will respect her privacy and do everything possible to maintain her modesty in the perioperative period.

Many GYN cases can be accomplished with epidural or intrathecal anesthesia, but few patients will desire a regional approach. If the patient is healthy and wants to go to sleep, we generally don't argue. We save our arm twisting for the morbidly obese patient or the patient with an unusual medical condition, and even then we usually have to promise to provide generous sedation once the block is in.

One other factor that tends to lead us away from regional anesthesia is the growing use of the laparoscope in GYN surgery. Even cases that were once guaranteed to stay out of the peritoneum, like vaginal hysterectomies, are now commonly done with a laparoscope "assist." And short cases, like ovarian cyst resections or appendectomies, may now be prolonged by the preliminary use of the scope. (The surgeon does this with a reason: If the patient's abdominal pain turns out to be from a nonoperable cause, the patient is spared a big incision.)

Many times the whole operation can be done through the scope, a trend we expect to see broadening as equipment improves and insurance companies get tougher.

What you get out of the GYN service: a few regional procedures, with deep sedation; a few mask cases; and a whole pile of straightforward general anesthetics in healthy patients. This is a good service for you to learn about different relaxants or narcotics, or try different techniques. Push yourself a little!

Dilatation and Curettage (D&C)

Description: The surgeon places a weighted speculum to allow a clear view of the cervix, then dilates the cervix with a series of progressively larger blunt probes. Once the cervical os is open, a series of scraping instruments (or a vacuum scraper) are inserted to remove the uterine mucosa.

Position:	Lithotomy
Estimated time:	30 minutes
Estimated blood loss:	200 ml; type and screen
Need for muscle relaxation:	Helpful
Indicated monitors:	Standard
Postoperative analgesia:	II
Acceptable techniques:	Local (paracervical block), GETA, spinal, MAC

Comments: The patient may be a healthy young woman who has suffered a miscarriage, in which case the D&C is performed to make sure there are no retained portions of placenta, or an older woman with dysfunctional uterine bleeding, in which case a sample of uterine mucosa is needed for biopsy. In either case the patient is apt to be very nervous and may need a fair amount of sedation.

Pregnant patients are much more sensitive to anesthetics than nonpregnant patients and are at increased risk for aspirating if given a general anesthetic. These patients should be steered toward a spinal or paracervical block.

Nonpregnant patients who have been NPO can be managed with a mask general anesthetic.

Oxytocin (Pitocin) and even methylergonovine maleate (Methergine) may be needed to slow uterine bleeding after a miscarriage. Make sure you have some on hand. Really persistent bleeding should make you—and the surgeon—think about a uterine perforation.

Cervical Cone Biopsy (LEEP, CKC)

Description: In response to an abnormal Pap smear, the surgeon goes in and resects the offending portion of the cervix.

Position:	Lithotomy
Estimated time:	45 minutes
Estimated blood loss:	100 ml; type and screen
Need for muscle relaxation:	Helpful
Indicated monitors:	Standard
Postoperative analgesia:	II
Acceptable techniques:	GA, spinal, epidural

Comments: The patients are usually young and otherwise healthy but may be nervous about the outcome of the biopsy.

CKC stands for cold knife conization. We can never remember what LEEP stands for, except that the *L* is for laser. Basically, it's two different ways of accomplishing the same thing. If a laser is involved you will of course want to refer to the appropriate section in Chapter 1.

Control of bleeding is typically the crux of the operation for the surgeon. Injection of a dilute local anesthetic solution containing epinephrine will commonly precede the resection, and this can help. Otherwise there's nothing to be done except cauterize and suture until things are under control. This occasionally becomes a tedious process for all concerned.

Rarely, cervical manipulation can cause bradycardia in the lightly anesthetized patient. Be prepared!

Tubal Ligation

Description: The surgeon makes a small transverse abdominal incision, reaches into the peritoneum, pulls out a fallopian tube, and ligates it. Same with the other tube. Closes the incision. Alternatively, the surgeon can do a laparoscopy and use a banding instrument to do the same thing percutaneously.

Position:	Supine, Trendelenburg for a laparoscopy
Estimated time:	30 minutes
Estimated blood loss:	Minimal; type and screen
Need for muscle relaxation:	Helpful
Indicated monitors:	Standard
Postoperative analgesia:	II
Acceptable techniques:	Spinal, epidural, GA

Comments: Always young, usually healthy patients. A fair percentage may be within a day or two of their last pregnancy, which can complicate your anesthetic.

When done via a minilaparotomy, virtually any anesthetic technique can be used. Postoperative pain is usually minimal.

When done laparoscopically, GETA is usually preferred, as abdominal distension is poorly tolerated by the awake patient. The usual laparoscopy concerns apply (see Chapter 1). Banding the tubes through a laparoscope may be more painful postoperatively than ligating them, due perhaps to ischemia of the crushed tube.

When performed on the recent parturient, bear in mind that the patient may still be at risk for aspiration from a general anesthetic and will still be exquisitely sensitive to most anesthetic agents. Use doses appropriate for a pregnant patient and you'll do fine.

Diagnostic Laparoscopy

Description: The surgeon makes a small incision in the umbilicus and introduces a trocar into the peritoneum. The belly is distended with CO_2, and a laparoscope attached to a camera is introduced for a look around. Additional entry ports to the peritoneum can be placed as needed to insert a variety of graspers, pluckers, buzzers, cutters, and other instruments. Endometrial implants can be resected (sometimes vaporized with a laser). Ovarian cysts can be resected, adhesions can be lysed, and the fallopian tubes can be manipulated.

Position:	Supine, Trendelenburg, sometimes low stirrups
Estimated time:	60 minutes
Estimated blood loss:	Minimal; type and screen
Need for muscle relaxation:	Required
Indicated monitors:	Standard
Postoperative analgesia:	II
Acceptable techniques:	GETA, spinal

Comments: The patients are usually young and seldom have a lot of other medical problems. Because of the technical difficulties involved, the surgeon will seldom bring an extremely overweight patient to the OR for a diagnostic scope.

Postoperative pain is a function of what the surgeon does. A great deal of resection or tissue manipulation or the cauterization of several endometriomas will make the patient very sore afterwards. A simple look around, on the other hand, will scarcely slow them down.

Postoperative nausea and vomiting are common enough in this population to make intraoperative prophylaxis a strong consideration.

Although your more stoic individuals will tolerate a laparoscopy under spinal anesthesia, it won't be any walk in the park. Abdominal distension and the Trendelenburg position will both make breathing difficult. This option should only be extended to very highly motivated patients.

End-tidal CO_2 will invariably rise during laparoscopy, due to absorption from the peritoneum. We mostly ignore it as long as the patient is hemodynamically stable.

See also the section on laparoscopy in Chapter 1.

Total Abdominal Hysterectomy (TAH)

Description: Through an abdominal incision, either transverse (at the "bikini line") or up and down, the surgeon accesses the peritoneum. After a brief exploration of the rest of the belly, the uterus and sometimes ovaries are separated from their blood supply and removed. The abdomen is then closed.

Position:	Supine
Estimated time:	3 hours
Estimated blood loss:	400 ml; type and cross-match 2 units
Need for muscle relaxation:	Required
Indicated monitors:	Standard, Foley, consider an A-line
Postoperative analgesia:	III
Acceptable techniques:	GETA, combined

Comments: The patient can be any age and may be anywhere from very healthy to very sick. Some hysterectomies are done for benign disease: uterine fibroids, excessive prolapse, or dysfunctional bleeding. These are usually the easy ones, on the short end of the time and blood-loss estimates.

Some hysterectomies are done for uterine or ovarian cancer, and these are often horrendous. A radical resection may include the omentum, the appendix, and a variety of lymph nodes and may take all day and several units of blood to complete. These are the patients who need arterial lines.

The structures most at risk of collateral damage during a TAH are the ureters. Pay close attention to urine output throughout the case, and report any sudden drop off in volume or change in color to the surgeon. (The surgeon will tell you the urine is red because of bladder manipulation, and most of the time that will be the case. Most of the time.)

Cancer patients may be very sick beforehand, both physically and psychologically. The patient with ascites will have a very rocky perioperative course, characterized by extreme fluid shifts, and may require pulmonary artery catheterization, frequent blood sampling, and postoperative intensive care.

Significant heat loss is common during hysterectomies. Be aggressive in keeping the patient warm: use a blood warmer, an active or passive airway heater, and as much upper body insulation as you can find.

Total Vaginal Hysterectomy (TVH)

Description: We're not exactly sure how this operation is done, since normally only the surgeon has any kind of view. We know that it involves incising around the cervix and pulling the uterus down and out, while ligating the vessels on either side, but it can be hard to follow any more closely than that.

Position:	Lithotomy
Estimated time:	3 hours
Estimated blood loss:	500 ml; type and cross-match 2 units
Need for muscle relaxation:	Helpful
Indicated monitors:	Standard
Postoperative analgesia:	II
Acceptable techniques:	GETA, spinal, epidural

Comments: Usually these patients are healthy, with a nonmalignant diagnosis, since this technique allows for no examination of the peritoneum or biopsy sampling of nearby tissues.

We've met some surgeons who could do this procedure a lot faster than 3 hours, but these were folks who had done hundreds of them. Most resident gynecologists will take a good deal longer, and will take a long time to get faster at it (probably *because* only the operating surgeon can see what's going on).

Nowadays this operation can be done with a laparoscopic assist, in which a diagnostic laparoscopy is done first to look around the peritoneum, free up any obvious adhesions, and do some of the dissecting of the uterus. This approach usually adds an hour or so to the length of the procedure but may help reduce the blood loss and avoid unpleasant surprises. See the section on diagnostic laparoscopy in this chapter and the discussion of laparoscopy in Chapter 1 for more information.

You have good access to the patient's airway, so it's not unreasonable to start the case with a regional anesthetic. If the surgery goes quickly you may even get away with it for the whole case.

In nonlaparoscopic TVHs, beware of the patient who has had previous abdominal surgery. Scar tissue and adhesions may make an all-day epic out of the case.

In the nonlaparoscopic vaginal hysterectomy, the possibility for occult intraperitoneal bleeding exists, as well as injury to one or both of the patient's ureters. Pay attention to the vital signs and the urine output in the PACU, and don't be afraid to call the surgeon back for a look if the patient seems to be unstable.

Bladder Suspension

Description: After carrying a baby or two, the pelvic floor begins to sag a little bit, the anatomic relationship of the bladder and urethra is distorted, and the patient starts to leak urine at embarrassing moments. There are a variety of surgeries to correct this problem (Marshall-Marchetti-Krantz [MMK], anterior and/or posterior repair, etc.), presenting to you under a variety of different names. They all have a similar purpose, though: to resuspend the bladder so that it no longer leaks under stress.

Position:	Lithotomy or low stirrups
Estimated time:	90 minutes
Estimated blood loss:	200 ml; type and screen
Need for muscle relaxation:	Helpful
Indicated monitors:	Standard
Postoperative analgesia:	II
Acceptable techniques:	GETA, spinal, epidural

Comments: The patients are usually embarrassed mothers in otherwise good health.

Although a small lower abdominal incision is often part of the case, there is minimal stimulation of the peritoneum or its contents, so that regional anesthesia is usually well tolerated. Most of these women will have had epidurals during childbirth.

The surgeon will be very interested in hearing about the patient's urinary output postoperatively, especially if there isn't any. It's possible to get the bladder-urethra junction too tight or to bag the ureters during the surgery, either of which will result in a complete obstruction of urine flow and an early return to the OR.

Tubal Anastomosis

Description: Through a transverse lower abdominal incision, the surgeon finds the loose ends of each fallopian tube, establishes their patency, and then, using a microscope, reconnects them.

Position:	Supine
Estimated time:	3 hours
Estimated blood loss:	100 ml; type and screen
Need for muscle relaxation:	Required
Indicated monitors:	Standard
Postoperative analgesia:	III
Acceptable techniques:	GETA, combined

Comments: Your population will be young, healthy patients who are eager to have children.

Don't let the patient move during the microsurgery portion of the case, as this will delay things substantially while the surgeon yells at you.

In this patient population a combined epidural and general anesthetic does not convey any greater safety intraoperatively, but it may help with postoperative pain if your hospital is set up to handle epidural infusions.

Cystectomy/Oophorectomy

Description: Through a small lower abdominal incision, the surgeon finds the ovarian mass and removes it. Sometimes this involves just the cyst; sometimes this means the whole ovary.

Position:	Supine
Estimated time:	2 hours
Estimated blood loss:	100 ml; type and screen
Need for muscle relaxation:	Required
Indicated monitors:	Standard
Postoperative analgesia:	III
Acceptable techniques:	GETA, combined

Comments: This operation may come up in women of any age but is most common in 20- to 40-year-olds. The patient is usually healthy otherwise but may be extremely nervous about the possibility that the mass is cancerous.

Ovarian cancer, by the way, usually necessitates the complete removal of the uterus, ovaries, omentum, appendix, and any handy lymph nodes, and is a very big ugly deal, so the patient has reason to be nervous.

Simple ovarian cysts can now be resected laparoscopically, and most operations will start this way in the hope they can finish this way as well. See the section on diagnostic laparoscopy in this chapter as well as the laparoscopy section in Chapter 1.

If laparoscopy looks likely, you should just stick to a GETA, since an epidural will be a bit of overkill.

Very motivated patients can handle lower abdominal incisions under regional (spinal or epidural) anesthesia, but you should be ready to deal with pain on manipulation of upper abdominal organs, nausea and vomiting from peritoneal stimulation, and apnea from a high block. Regional anesthesia is even less suited to laparoscopic surgery because of the added annoyance of abdominal distension and Trendelenburg positioning.

In Vitro Fertilization

Description: In a miracle of modern medical technology, a ripe egg is identified in the patient's ovary via transabdominal or transvaginal ultrasound and then sucked out with a fine needle. If there are many ripe eggs (usually there are if the patient is on fertility drugs), as many are sucked out as possible. Meanwhile, in a nearby room the husband is donating "the gift," as it is euphemistically called. Egg and sperm are then invited to meet in a test tube, and the resulting zygote is implanted back in the uterus using some variation on a turkey baster.

Position:	Lithotomy
Estimated time:	60 minutes
Estimated blood loss:	Minimal
Need for muscle relaxation:	None
Indicated monitors:	Standard
Postoperative analgesia:	I
Acceptable techniques:	Spinal, epidural, GA, MAC, local

Comments: The patients are healthy and have usually been trying to get pregnant for ages. They may have been summoned for the procedure on a moment's notice, when the gynecologist decided that the developing eggs were just right.

There are various theories about which anesthetics are good for this procedure. From our point of view it's no big deal. Fine-needle aspiration of the ovary is uncomfortable, sure, but it's not like having a kidney removed. Your problems will come from the infertility surgeon, who may feel that one sort of anesthesia is worse for the harvested egg than another. We mostly do these with a low-dose lidocaine spinal, although other possibilities include mask general, MAC, or don't-call-us-at-all. Check with the surgeon on this.

Obstetrics

The key to understanding anesthesia for pregnant women is having a good grasp of the normal physiologic changes of pregnancy. As follows:

1. A smaller functional residual capacity (FRC) and an increased oxygen consumption limit the parturient's ability to tolerate prolonged apnea. Desaturation will begin within 90 seconds of the cessation of breathing.

2. Edema of the oronasopharynx is universal. In the presence of pre-eclampsia it can be even more pronounced. Plan on using a smaller than usual endotracheal tube (6.0–7.0), and avoid putting anything in the nose. Optimize the patient's head position before starting.

3. Decreased FRC and increased minute ventilation lead to rapid uptake of volatile anesthetics.

4. Aortocaval compression (see Fig. 1-10) can occur as early as the twentieth week of gestation and will cause decreased preload and a resulting fall in blood pressure. Any time the patient is supine, you should provide left uterine displacement by putting a bump under the right hip.

5. Gastric volumes increase in pregnancy, gastric pH decreases, intestinal motility falls, and the lower esophageal sphincter weakens, all of which put the patient at greatly increased risk for reflux and aspiration during general anesthesia. All inductions should be either awake or rapid sequence.

6. Total circulating protein, including albumin, drops during pregnancy, increasing the free fraction of some drugs. At the same time fat and free water are increasing, increasing the volume of distribution of many drugs and potentially changing half-lives. Paradoxically, the pregnant patient has a significantly greater response to anesthetics than the nonpregnant patient, minimal alveolar concentration is 40% lower, and initial IV doses should be halved.

7. Pregnant patients are also dramatically more sensitive to local anesthetics. Normal epidural and spinal

doses will produce higher levels and longer durations than in nonpregnant patients. This effect may be due to a smaller epidural/intrathecal space or secondary to engorged epidural veins, as well as to a primary effect of progesterone on the nerves.

8. Cardiac output is higher, plasma volume is higher, red cell mass is higher, but hematocrit is lower (plasma volume rises more than red cell mass). Blood is lost at delivery, and diuresis occurs shortly thereafter to return the patient to a euvolemic state.

9. Lower extremity edema is normal and probably relates to venous obstruction by the gravid uterus. Edema above the knees is not normal, however, and may be a sign of pre-eclampsia.

There is a great deal more we could say about the normal course of labor and delivery, fetal monitoring, and common obstetric diseases like pre-eclampsia or gestational diabetes, but we only have so much space. We refer you now to the case presentations.

Dilatation and Curettage (D&C)

Description: The surgeon places a weighted speculum to allow a clear view of the cervix, then dilates it with a series of progressively larger blunt probes. Once the cervical os is open, a series of scraping instruments (or a vacuum scraper) are inserted to remove the uterine mucosa.

Position:	Lithotomy
Estimated time:	30 minutes
Estimated blood loss:	200 ml; type and screen
Need for muscle relaxation:	Helpful
Indicated monitors:	Standard
Postoperative analgesia:	II
Acceptable techniques:	Local (paracervical block), GETA, spinal, MAC

Comments: The patient may be a healthy young woman who has suffered a miscarriage, in which case the D&C is performed to make sure there are no retained portions of placenta, or an older woman with dysfunctional uterine bleeding, in which case a sample of uterine mucosa is needed for biopsy. In either case the patient is apt to be very nervous and may need a fair amount of sedation.

Pregnant patients are much more sensitive to anesthetics than nonpregnant patients and are at increased risk for aspirating if given a general anesthetic. These patients should be steered toward a spinal or paracervical block.

Nonpregnant patients who have been NPO can be managed with a mask general anesthetic.

Oxytocin (Pitocin) and even methylergonovine maleate (Methergine) may be needed to slow uterine bleeding after a miscarriage. Make sure you have some on hand. Really persistent bleeding should make you—and the surgeon—think about a uterine perforation.

Vaginal Delivery

Description: Unlike most procedures, this one is performed primarily by the patient. The surgeon's participation consists of performing an episiotomy (if needed) to help prevent tearing of the perineum, or deciding that a forceps or C-section delivery is indicated. Otherwise the mom does all the hard work.

Position:	Lithotomy
Estimated time:	Indefinite
Estimated blood loss:	300 ml; type and screen
Need for muscle relaxation:	Contraindicated
Indicated monitors:	As needed
Postoperative analgesia:	II
Acceptable techniques:	None, local, spinal, epidural

Comments: The patient will generally be in good health, although "terminally pregnant." It is important for you to understand the normal physiologic changes of pregnancy, summarized in the beginning of this chapter.

Anesthesia may not be required at all for a vaginal delivery, but in these civilized times it is often preferred. Local to the perineum is indicated if an episiotomy is being performed (something the surgeon will take care of). For a patient close to delivery who needs a more serious anesthetic, or for the postpartum patient with a complex perineal laceration to repair, a "saddle block" is the best bet. This means a low spinal, done with a hyperbaric solution with the patient sitting up, so that only the lowest nerve roots get anesthetized. The antepartum patient should still be able to sense her contractions and push to deliver the baby.

For the patient confronting an indeterminate amount of labor, the recommended approach is an epidural, dosed to achieve analgesia but not complete anesthesia, and maintained with either repeated reinjections or a continuous infusion. For perinatal perineal pain or a C-section, a denser block can be established.

Monitoring should be limited to what is situationally relevant, so as not to get in the way. The awake patient with a working epidural analgesic only needs an anesthesiologist somewhere in the building. A dense block achieved by spinal or epidural requires you to be in attendance, so that you can decide which other monitors are needed. Blood pressure measurement every so often is a good idea and won't usually get in the way. Oximetry and ECG monitoring are nice but tend to get tangled and disconnected while the patient pushes and are not commonly used with healthy laboring parturients. An intermittent signal is about the best you can hope for.

Watch the fetal heart recording and learn to interpret it. Fetal distress (i.e., bradycardia) is best managed initially with oxygen, support of the blood pressure, and repositioning of the patient. Get the nurse to help!

Oxytocin (Pitocin) (10–20 units) is added to the IV after the placenta is delivered.

Remember to keep the patient's right hip bumped up to provide left uterine displacement whenever the patient is lying flat.

Cesarean Section (C-Section)

Description: The surgeon makes a transverse incision through the lower abdominal wall and lower uterine segment, reaches into the uterus and delivers the baby, removes the placenta, and closes.

Position:	Supine, left uterine displacement
Estimated time:	60 minutes
Estimated blood loss:	700 ml; type and screen
Need for muscle relaxation:	Required
Indicated monitors:	Standard, Foley to get bladder out of the way
Postoperative analgesia:	III
Acceptable techniques:	GETA, spinal, epidural

Comments: The patients are usually young and healthy, with one of a variety of indications for surgical delivery: fetal distress, cephalopelvic disproportion, failure to progress, impending chorioamnionitis, previous C-sections, twins, or the like. Some of these indications are urgent, some are semi-urgent, and some are elective. Ask the obstetrician if you don't know.

Regional anesthesia is preferred in all but the most urgent cases (bleeding, severe fetal distress) to allow Mom to be awake for the delivery and to avoid a potentially bad airway in a patient with high aspiration risk. You may be able to continue the anesthetic that is already in place. If GETA is indicated, this must be done either in a rapid-sequence fashion with cricoid pressure (more common) or awake (less common).

The estimated blood loss averages 1,000 ml, but most of it is unneeded by the mother once the baby has been delivered. The important question for you to ask, once the placenta is out, is "Is the uterus contracting down adequately?" If yes, then the bleeding will stop as the uterus is closed. If no, then you need to know about it sooner rather than later. Oxytocin (Pitocin) (10–20 units) is added to the IV infusion as soon as the placenta is delivered. Run this in slowly, or you will aggravate any hypotension your anesthetic has already caused. Oxytocin administration may also cause flushing and a headache. Methylergonovine maleate (Methergine), when indicated to control uterine bleeding, is given IM, not IV.

Remember that your primary responsibility is to the mother, not the baby.

Many surgeons will ask for antibiotics to be given after the baby is delivered.

The patient will be very sensitive to any anesthetic, particularly if she has had a long and arduous labor. Plan on starting with half the dose that you would give a nonpregnant patient and see what happens before giving any more. A small dose of midazolam (0.5 mg) may make the patient completely somnolent!

Nausea and vomiting are common, as is shivering. Keep the blood pressure up, keep the patient wrapped up, and provide reassurance as necessary. Nausea may be your first sign of hypotension.

Forceps/Vacuum Delivery

Description: Once in a while the baby gets stuck close to delivery and needs a little help. Forceps are used to guide the baby out of the birth canal, provide a little bit of positive pull, and maintain progress between contractions. A vacuum extractor serves basically the same purpose in a different way. The mother is still required to do most of the pushing.

Position:	Lithotomy
Estimated time:	30 minutes
Estimated blood loss:	400 ml; type and screen
Need for muscle relaxation:	Contraindicated
Indicated monitors:	Standard
Postoperative analgesia:	II
Acceptable techniques:	Epidural, spinal

Comments: The patient is the usual healthy pregnant woman but may be worn out from pushing for several hours against an uncooperative pelvis. She will be looking forward to a little pain relief but will be anxious about the use of forceps or the vacuum extractor.

We figure the up-front odds of going to a C-section at about 50% whenever the surgeon picks up the forceps. (Obstetricians will quote you much lower numbers, of course, but we're talking about the training environment here. The use of forceps is a difficult skill that takes years to learn.) Your choice of an anesthetic should take this into account, especially since some of the C-sections will be on an emergent basis. We generally prefer to approach a forceps delivery with an epidural level of about T-8 to T-10: high enough to cut on right away if a disaster occurs, but low enough that the patient will still be able to push effectively with some good coaching. You should be prepared to put your hand on her belly and tell her when she is having a contraction, so that she can push. If you do this smoothly enough, the obstetrician will never notice that the patient is too numb to feel anything.

In the absence of an epidural, a spinal can be used for anesthesia, but make sure you discuss it with the obstetrician first. If he or she swears that the baby will deliver with low forceps and that a C-section is unlikely, then you can try and keep the level low enough for the patient to push. This may result in an emergent general anesthetic, though, which will put the mother at risk for aspiration and failure to intubate. Take a good look at the airway before agreeing to do a low spinal!

Oxygen is a good idea, and whatever standard monitors you can get to stay on with the patient pushing. Keep an eye on the fetal monitor and remember to provide left uterine displacement whenever the patient is lying flat.

Cerclage Placement

Description: The surgeon takes a big ol' suture and runs it around the cervix in a purse string, then pulls it tight. With luck, it keeps the oven door closed until the cooking is done.

Position:	Lithotomy
Estimated time:	30 minutes
Estimated blood loss:	Minimal
Need for muscle relaxation:	Helpful
Indicated monitors:	Standard, fetal monitoring
Postoperative analgesia:	I
Acceptable techniques:	Spinal, GETA, epidural, paracervical block

Comments: This procedure is done on otherwise healthy pregnant patients with a history of premature cervical dilatation and spontaneous abortion. The cerclage is usually placed at about 20 weeks, as the uterus is just getting big enough to be a problem. Check out the physiologic changes of pregnancy before starting!

A spinal or paracervical block will be the quickest and easiest way to go. General anesthesia necessitates intubation, because of the increased risk of aspiration in the pregnant patient, and may expose the fetus to drugs such as N_2O and benzodiazepines, which are potentially harmful.

Talk to the obstetrician before the procedure and decide whether the fetus is viable or not. If yes, then continuous fetal monitoring is probably a good idea; one complication of the procedure is premature rupture of the membranes and subsequent delivery. If the fetus is not viable (and at 20 weeks, it isn't), the patient should be aware of this in advance so that if a miscarriage is induced, the necessary psychological and medicolegal groundwork has been laid.

The cerclage, if effective, will be removed when the fetus is sufficiently mature to be delivered. Cerclage removal can usually be accomplished without anesthesia or with a local block, but occasionally a real anesthetic is required. If the patient is already laboring or expected to deliver soon after the cerclage is removed, it might be a good time to put in an epidural.

Gravid Hysterectomy

Description: The surgeon makes an incision as for a C-section (but often in a bigger hurry), delivers the baby, and then proceeds to ligate the uterine arteries, tie off and separate the ligaments supporting the uterus, and remove the specimen. The ovaries may or may not be included.

Position:	Supine, left uterine displacement
Estimated time:	4 hours
Estimated blood loss:	1,500 ml plus; type and crossmatch 6 units
Need for muscle relaxation:	Required
Indicated monitors:	Standard, Foley, A-line; consider CVP line
Postoperative analgesia:	III
Acceptable techniques:	GETA, combined

Comments: This procedure is seldom a planned event but occurs as the result of a uterine rupture during labor (in which case the baby is often dead); a placenta accreta (in which case the baby has usually already been delivered); a flaccid, bleeding uterus; or some other misadventure during a C-section. The patient usually begins the operation healthy but pregnant, but may already have lost a large volume of blood by the time the hysterectomy starts.

This case will be a bloodbath. Don't give up the ship! Be prepared to transfuse large amounts of warmed fluid (i.e., have plenty of good IV access), and go to fresh-frozen plasma and platelets early. Disseminated intravascular coagulation is common but in the otherwise healthy patient can be overcome if you just stay on top of it.

If you are using an epidural alone, you should induce general anesthesia as soon as you realize that something's up. You can continue to use the epidural for the bulk of your anesthetic unless you start to run into problems with the patient's blood pressure; a sympathectomy will make your life slightly more difficult but may actually reduce bleeding overall. It's a good idea to secure the airway before hanging 50 units of blood, though.

Yes, 50. And we've seen it go even higher—in patients who survived without complication.

Think hard before extubating the patient at the end of the case. Just how much airway edema is there? Consider a leak test or direct laryngoscopy prior to extubation.

Sudden pulmonary dysfunction can result from autoimmune reactions to embolized amniotic fluid or from transfused blood. Treat this with epinephrine and cross your fingers.

Orthopedic Surgery

To be an orthopedic surgeon, you need to have been one of those kids who enjoyed messing around in Dad's workshop, playing with the power tools. The joke is that you must be the sort who would have been a fine carpenter, but thought you'd go to medical school to learn a trade—either that, or a smart ex-jock.

Orthopedic surgery involves diagnosis and repair of all the skeletal bones and joints from the foramen magnum down. This can range from simple closed repairs of forearm fractures all the way up to straightening a severely curved spine. In academic centers, orthopedic departments divide themselves into a variety of subservices: general (acute fractures and trauma), sports-related, joint replacement, hands and feet, pediatric, and spine. In the community these distinctions are largely forgotten, and one lucky doctor will do it all.

Orthopedic patients can run the gamut from young children with cerebral palsy and joint contractures to nonagenarians with Alzheimer's disease and fractured hips. Trauma is a common cause of the patient's problem, and associated injuries and severe pain are not unusual preoperatively. Other than that, though, orthopedic patients are often healthy and active folk who are willing to indulge your interest in regional anesthesia.

Rapid blood loss is common in many orthopedic procedures. In other cases bleeding is controlled by a tourniquet during the important parts of the procedure. (Tourniquets are interesting enough in their own right that we have included a separate section on them, following this one.) Good IV access is important, as well as a sense of what the surgeons have done and what they still have left to do.

Starting and stopping an orthopedic case can be a time-consuming process. Positioning for surgery can be complex, often involving special tables with special attachments, some not commonly used since the height of the Inquisition. And at the end of the case, just when you're all ready to pull the tube and head for the golf course, the surgeon announces that he will need an extra half-hour for his elaborate dressing and cast placement and can you please keep the patient from moving, thank you very much.

Postoperative pain can be fairly intense following orthopedic surgery and will allow you to use all the blocks, infusions, and adjuvant modalities your heart desires. And the surgeons will be happy to see you do it, as long as the patient makes it to physical therapy on time.

TOURNIQUETS

One of the unique features of orthopedic surgery is the use of a tourniquet to reduce bleeding in the operative extremity. The tourniquet will typically be applied while the limb is being prepped and then inflated as needed later in the case. Here are some tips for tourniquet use:

1. Understand how the tourniquet goes on and how the inflation box works. Most tourniquets inflate with either compressed nitrogen or compressed air to a fixed pressure that can be set on the box. It is important to keep the tourniquet connected to the gas source throughout its use.

2. Pad under the tourniquet with cotton batting, and make sure it lies smoothly on the skin. Otherwise erythema and even skin sloughing can occur.

3. Preset the desired pressure on the inflation box. This should be approximately 100 mm Hg above the patient's mean systolic pressure—about 250 mm Hg for arms and 300 mm Hg for legs.

4. Turn the tourniquet on and it will inflate to the preset pressure. Have the surgeon bang it once or twice and watch for the pressure gauge needle to quiver. This "bounce test" tells you that the tourniquet and inflation box are working appropriately, and that you are not being suckered by a stuck gauge.

5. Write down the inflation time and pressure on your anesthetic record. Notify the surgeon at 60, 90, and 120 minutes after inflation. Leaving the tourniquet inflated beyond 120 minutes risks permanent damage to the limb.

6. After about an hour, most patients will begin to

experience "tourniquet pain," a nonspecific discomfort in the region of the tourniquet, often accompanied by progressive hypertension. In the anesthetized patient, you may see an impressive rise in anesthetic requirements (or the need for beta blockers), which can lead to a significant delay in waking the patient up, since tourniquet pain and hypertension vanish almost immediately with release of the pressure and reperfusion of the limb.

7. Tourniquet pain may be somewhat blunted by infiltration of the skin beneath the tourniquet site with local anesthetics (prior to putting the tourniquet on) or by regional anesthetics. But be aware that tourniquet pain and reflex hypertension can still occur even in the face of the densest spinal anesthetic.

8. Release of the tourniquet pressure, besides relieving tourniquet pain, will cause a transient systemic hypotension, a drop in core temperature (sometimes a rise, in pediatric cases), a rise in end-tidal carbon dioxide, and a noticeable metabolic acidosis. In most patients this effect is short-lived and clinically insignificant, but in those with marginal myocardial function it can cause an impressive dip.

9. Finally, should the surgeons desire to reinflate the tourniquet, make sure at least 10–20 minutes have elapsed before doing so. Even so, the washout of ischemic factors will not be complete, and tourniquet pain and acidosis will develop even more rapidly the second time.

Closed Reduction of Fracture/Relocation of Joint

Description: The surgeon straightens out the problem, using x-ray or fluoroscopy to verify that everything is back where it belongs.

Position:	As needed (most often supine)
Estimated time:	15 minutes
Estimated blood loss:	None
Need for muscle relaxation:	Helpful
Indicated monitors:	Standard
Postoperative analgesia:	II
Acceptable techniques:	GA, regional, MAC

Comments: Sometimes this procedure can be done under heavy sedation, using a benzodiazepine to confer some amount of muscle relaxation. This obviously works best with very short procedures, such as relocating a dislocated hip, knee, or shoulder.

This procedure tends to be an emergency, so full stomach considerations apply. Very heavy sedation or general anesthesia mandates an endotracheal tube.

Closed-fracture reductions, in particular, may become open procedures. Percutaneous pinning to secure the fracture counts as an open procedure and necessitates a serious regional or general anesthetic.

Frequent x-rays are common.

Don't forget to check the patient's secondary trauma assessment. Did she also hit her head when she fell? Avoid embarrassment and think carefully about the mechanism of injury before starting your anesthetic.

Open Reduction and Internal Fixation (ORIF) of the Wrist or Hand

Description: Through one or more small incisions, the bones of the hand are exposed, reduced, and held in the correct position by a series of small pins, plates, and screws.

Position:	Supine
Estimated time:	Variable
Estimated blood loss:	Minimal; type and screen
Need for muscle relaxation:	May be useful for the surgeons
Indicated monitors:	Standard, consider Foley
Postoperative analgesia:	II
Acceptable techniques:	GETA, axillary or supraclavicular block

Comments: If the patient's trauma is acute, treat the patient as if he or she has a full stomach and take a good look for additional injuries before starting. Consider whether the patient is drunk or otherwise impaired when planning your anesthetic.

No monitors or IVs on the surgical side!

The surgeon will place a tourniquet and may use it to control bleeding on the field. This can be one of those cases where it is inflated and deflated several times.

Expect frequent x-rays.

Regional anesthesia can be very effective and can be easily converted to general if the case goes long. Make sure you have discussed and documented all pre-existing neurologic deficits before sticking a needle anywhere near the brachial plexus.

At the end of the case there will be upwards of 30 minutes of elaborate wound dressing and casting. Don't wake the patient up too early.

Open Reduction and Internal Fixation (ORIF) of the Forearm

Description: The forearm is opened lengthwise, the broken bones are reduced, and plates and screws are used to hold things where they belong.

Position:	Supine
Estimated time:	2 hours
Estimated blood loss:	150 ml; type and cross-match 2 units
Need for muscle relaxation:	Helpful for the surgeon
Indicated monitors:	Standard, consider Foley
Postoperative analgesia:	II
Acceptable techniques:	GETA, upper extremity block

Comments: These are usually trauma patients and may have full stomachs and other injuries. Early surgery will generally be faster, because the surgeons will have less edema to deal with, but delaying surgery by 24–48 hours will not usually harm patients. It may also allow them to sober up.

No monitors or IVs on the operative side. Expect the surgeon to use a tourniquet.

Expect a certain amount of radiation exposure.

Although forearm fractures are usually pretty straightforward, any damage to the nerves or arteries will necessitate a microvascular repair and prolong the operation substantially. Make sure you have documented any neurovascular abnormalities on your record before initiating a regional anesthetic.

Allow time for cast construction before waking the patient up.

Open Reduction and Internal Fixation (ORIF) of the Humerus

Description: A longitudinal incision is made to expose the fracture site, traction is applied to reduce the bone, and it is then plated and screwed for stability.

Position:	Semi-Fowler's
Estimated time:	3 hours
Estimated blood loss:	500 ml; type and cross-match 2 units
Need for muscle relaxation:	Required for surgical reduction
Indicated monitors:	Standard, Foley
Postoperative analgesia:	III
Acceptable techniques:	GETA, can be combined with interscalene

Comments: These cases are almost always done acutely for trauma victims. The force required to fracture the humerus is substantial, and you should have a high index of suspicion for associated injuries. A rapid-sequence induction and aspiration prophylaxis are indicated—even more so if the patient is inebriated.

Damage to the neurovascular bundle is common in fractures of the humerus, and repairing this structure may be time-consuming. Make sure you have documented a thorough neurologic exam before initiating any sort of adjuvant regional anesthesia.

Needless to say (but we'll say it anyway), your lines and monitors should all be on the nonoperative extremity.

Stabilizing the humerus surgically can be quite challenging. The newer rodding systems used for the femur are mostly too large for the humerus, while plating systems may not be strong enough to resist muscular forces in the arm. Expect a longish case and a lot of radiation exposure from frequent use of the C-arm.

Open Reduction and Internal Fixation (ORIF) of the Foot or Ankle

Description: An appropriate incision is made to provide access to the fracture site, the bone fragments are reapproximated, and everything is held together with a collection of small plates and screws.

Position:	Supine, usually
Estimated time:	2 hours
Estimated blood loss:	200 ml; type and cross-match 2 units
Need for muscle relaxation:	Not necessary
Indicated monitors:	Standard
Postoperative analgesia:	II
Acceptable techniques:	GETA, spinal, epidural, leg block

Comments: These patients are usually young healthy trauma victims, typically without a lot of associated injuries (but ask anyway), but possibly with some ethanol on board. If the surgeon can get to the problem early, there will be less tissue edema and the procedure will go faster. This may mean doing a rapid-sequence intubation, if the patient is still thought to have a full stomach.

A tourniquet will typically be placed and used if bleeding becomes a problem.

Epidural anesthesia requires a fairly long set-up time for procedures at the ankle but does offer the advantage of being able to redose if things run long (although switching to general anesthesia is not a big deal). Any regional technique should be preceded by a careful neurologic exam of the affected extremity, so that everyone is clear later as to what defects existed before and which were created intra-op.

Expect a certain amount of fluoroscopy.

Open Reduction and Internal Fixation (ORIF) of the Femur

Description: A long lateral incision at the hip is combined with a small incision above the knee. A long metal rod is placed across the fracture and down the shaft of the femur, screws are used to secure it at each end, and the incisions are closed.

Position:	Supine on fracture table, leg in traction
Estimated time:	3 hours
Estimated blood loss:	500 ml plus; type and crossmatch 4 units
Need for muscle relaxation:	Required
Indicated monitors:	Standard, Foley, A-line; consider CVP line
Postoperative analgesia:	III
Acceptable techniques:	GETA, spinal, epidural, or combined

Comments: A large force (or a metastatic tumor) is required to fracture the femur. Secondary assessment for other injuries or disease states is very important. Consider aspiration prophylaxis and a rapid-sequence induction. Reduce your induction doses if the patient is already "anesthetized" (i.e., drunk).

This case can be complicated by substantial blood and heat loss. Be especially aware of your preoperative situation: Substantial blood loss can occur even in a closed femur fracture. Use a blood warmer and an active airway heater, and keep the patient as well covered as you can.

Pounding a steel rod down the femur creates an enormous rise in intramedullary pressure and may displace substantial amounts of fat, marrow, or tumor into the circulation. This in turn may trigger allergic reactions in the lung and elsewhere, leading to full-blown hemodynamic collapse. Epinephrine is the drug of choice for this syndrome and should be used early and often.

Patients presenting for rodding of the femur secondary to an existing or impending pathologic fracture are usually extremely poor surgical candidates. Tumor embolization is also much more likely to trigger a systemic reaction than fat or marrow, and the patient is less likely to tolerate the insult. Put in lots of lines (including a pulmonary artery catheter), and expect trouble.

A certain amount of intraoperative fluoroscopy is required to confirm correct placement of the hardware.

Hip Pinning

Description: In uncomplicated hip fractures, sometimes all that is required is a single large screw across the fracture site and a plate to secure it to the femur.

Position:	Supine, on fracture table, leg in traction
Estimated time:	60 minutes
Estimated blood loss:	200 ml; type and screen 2 units
Need for muscle relaxation:	Not necessary
Indicated monitors:	Standard
Postoperative analgesia:	II (minimal pain once the fracture is fixed)
Acceptable techniques:	GETA, spinal, epidural

Comments: The typical patient for a hip pinning is 85 years old, which tends to color the anesthetic approach. Even in those without Alzheimer's disease, very exaggerated responses to IV sedatives can be expected. Coexisting medical problems are common. Consideration must also be given to the mechanism of injury and the potential for undiscovered additional injuries. If the patient was down for a long time awaiting assistance, you can expect dehydration and even myoglobinuria to complicate your anesthetic.

The patient will be in significant pain until the hip is fixed. Sometimes a little fentanyl or ketamine is required, along with surgical assistance to maintain traction, when positioning the patient for a spinal or epidural.

The sympathectomy will hit hard, especially if you used the sedation recommended in the previous paragraph. Have your phenylephrine infusion ready, and turn it on early.

Expect a certain amount of fluoroscopy.

Most elderly patients will have very little pain once their fracture is reduced and stabilized. This can slow emergence from general anesthesia. Be cautious with your drug doses, use short-acting agents, and titrate carefully.

Bipolar Hip Replacement (Austin-Moore)

Description: In severe hip fractures, the surgeon simply removes the entire femoral head and replaces it with a steel prosthesis pounded into the proximal end of the femur.

Position:	Lateral decubitus
Estimated time:	150 minutes
Estimated blood loss:	500 ml; type and cross-match 2 units
Need for muscle relaxation:	Required for surgical exposure
Indicated monitors:	Standard, Foley; consider A-line
Postoperative analgesia:	III
Acceptable techniques:	GETA, spinal, epidural, or combined technique

Comments: This operation tends to be done in those patients with hip fractures who are likely to return to full function. They are usually a little less frail than the patients for hip pinning but may be both elderly and somewhat debilitated. Take a full history, especially looking for concurrent cardiac or pulmonary disease.

Consider the mechanism of injury and the potential for other occult trauma before anesthetizing the patient. Expect a full stomach, and plan on a rapid-sequence induction if using a general anesthetic.

Positioning the patient for a regional anesthetic can be quite painful. Sometimes a little bit of ketamine or fentanyl is necessary first, along with a cooperative assistant who can maintain traction on the fractured leg. While the patient is in traction (and once the hip is repaired) the pain is not usually too severe.

Pulmonary embolism of fat or marrow can occur with placement of the prosthesis and can be aggravated by the use of methylmethacrylate cement. Epinephrine is the drug of choice for hemodynamic instability, along with clean living and appropriate prayers.

Even without invoking embolic phenomena, methylmethacrylate cement (the unfixed monomer) can cause vasodilatation and hypotension. Be sure to have the patient well hydrated before the cement goes in.

Blood and heat loss can be substantial. Be prepared with good IV access, a fluid warmer, an active or passive airway warmer, and a warm OR.

Open Reduction and Internal Fixation (ORIF) of the Pelvis

Description: The fractured areas of the pelvis are exposed and may be fixed with plates and screws. An external fixator can also be used to hold the entire pelvic ring rigid; this device looks like an erector set hooked to long pins driven through various portions of the pelvic bone and requires a substantial amount of time and dissection to set up.

Position:	Supine; may require turning intraoperatively
Estimated time:	6 hours
Estimated blood loss:	1,000 ml; type and cross-match 6 units
Need for muscle relaxation:	Helpful for surgical exposure and manipulation
Indicated monitors:	Standard, Foley (careful!), A-line
Postoperative analgesia:	III
Acceptable techniques:	GETA, combined

Comments: Although these patients are customarily the young, healthy victims of high-speed automobile accidents, the mechanism of injury dictates a substantial degree of associated trauma, including disrupted abdominal viscera, fractured ribs, contused lungs, and closed head injuries. Very often, in fact, definitive repair of the pelvis will be delayed several days until other problems have been taken care of (and the patient sobers up).

Difficulty placing the Foley catheter is a red flag for urethral disruption. Call the urologist early if you have any problems.

Bleeding is usually the biggest concern and is the principal motivator for early repairs. Pelvic fractures can ooze forever, with no real way for the surgeons to control it other than by fixing the bone. Make sure your IV access is abundant, keep the patient warm, and notify the blood bank that they will be in for a long night. Give coagulation factors and platelets early if things are looking ugly. Read the section on blood loss in Chapter 1.

If or when the operative repair has been delayed long enough to make the patient hemodynamically stable, an epidural catheter is a reasonable way to reduce blood loss, minimize the risk of deep venous thrombosis formation, and manage postoperative pain. Positioning for the catheter placement can be difficult, though, and you will want to be careful with your sympathectomy in the face of severe bleeding. You may also want to find out if the patient has been anticoagulated before sticking anything in the back.

Expect a fair amount of fluoroscopy with the external fixation procedure.

Knee Arthroscopy

Description: The surgeon makes a small hole in the knee joint and sticks a fiberoptic scope/camera in it. The knee is distended by a continuous inflow of saline, and the surgeon is able to look at the full extent of the joint space. Various grabbers, shavers, and burrs (introduced through additional holes) can be used to remove redundant tissue, torn menisci, or bone spurs.

Position:	Supine
Estimated time:	60 minutes
Estimated blood loss:	Minimal; type and screen
Need for muscle relaxation:	Not required but may help with surgical manipulation
Indicated monitors:	Standard
Postoperative analgesia:	II
Acceptable techniques:	GA, spinal, epidural, leg block, local/MAC

Comments: Virtually any anesthetic technique can be used successfully, depending on the surgeon and the patient. Fast operations are most quickly done with GA by mask and/or local infiltration by the surgeon. In a training environment, regional or GETA is probably better.

A tourniquet is applied and may be inflated to reduce bleeding and improve visibility in the joint space. Tourniquet times are usually short. (See the discussion of tourniquets at the beginning of this chapter.)

Some surgeons will infiltrate the joint space with bupivacaine and/or morphine at the end of the procedure, making it essentially pain-free postoperatively. This can slow the patient's emergence from anesthesia if you are unprepared for it, especially because the case can end quite suddenly.

If the procedure runs long, the floor gets really wet from the irrigating fluid. Wear your waders!

Shoulder Arthroscopy

Description: An access port is opened in the shoulder joint, which is then distended with saline irrigation and examined with a fiberoptic scope attached to a camera. Other ports can be created for other instruments, allowing a certain amount of surgery without opening the joint space completely.

Position:	Semi-Fowler's, with the operative arm suspended from the ceiling
Estimated time:	2 hours
Estimated blood loss:	Minimal; type and screen
Need for muscle relaxation:	Very helpful for joint manipulation
Indicated monitors:	Standard
Postoperative analgesia:	II
Acceptable techniques:	GETA, interscalene block, or a combination

Comments: No IVs or monitors on the operative side, please.

You will have less access than you might like to the patient's airway once the case starts. This is an argument for combining your interscalene block with a GETA, and for securing your tube very carefully.

Bupivacaine and/or morphine injected into the joint space at the conclusion of the procedure will greatly minimize postoperative pain. Like all "-oscopies," this case can end quickly, so use the short-acting stuff.

Make sure you have returned the patient to a good position for reintubation before awakening and extubating.

Wrist/Ankle Arthroscopy

Description: A small hole is poked into the joint space, which is then distended with a gravity-powered saline infusion and examined with a fiberoptic scope connected to a camera. Other entry ports can be created for a variety of pokers, grabbers, and trimmers, although small joint arthroscopy is more commonly used for diagnostic purposes and less commonly intended to be operative.

Position:	Supine, with arm/foot elevated
Estimated time:	2 hours
Estimated blood loss:	Minimal
Need for muscle relaxation:	Not necessary
Indicated monitors:	Standard
Postoperative analgesia:	II
Acceptable techniques:	Wrist: GETA, axillary, or supraclavicular block; ankle: GETA, spinal, or leg block

Comments: Avoid putting any monitors or IVs on the operative extremity.

A tourniquet is usually placed preoperatively and may be used to limit bleeding.

Epidurals provide lousy anesthesia at the ankle (without a long set-up time), and wrist/ankle blocks are usually inadequate for the procedure.

Short-acting anesthetics are probably a good idea, since this case can end very quickly. One minute the surgeon will be working away in the joint space, providing maximal stimulation to the patient, and the next minute will be done. Closure involves no more than a few sutures.

Bupivacaine or morphine in the joint space at the end of the case will minimize postoperative pain, which also slows emergence.

Make the surgeon turn the monitor so that you can watch too. It'll help keep your attention on the procedure.

Anterior Cruciate Ligament Reconstruction

Description: Operating via a knee arthroscope, the surgeon drills holes in the femur and tibia, then threads a piece of tendon (usually harvested from the patellar tendon on the same side) through both holes, in place of the native anterior cruciate ligament. The tendon is attached to the bone on either side and, voilà, as good as new. Dr. Frankenstein would be proud.

Position:	Supine
Estimated time:	3 hours
Estimated blood loss:	Minimal; type and screen
Need for muscle relaxation:	Not necessary but may help surgical manipulation
Indicated monitors:	Standard, Foley
Postoperative analgesia:	III
Acceptable techniques:	GETA, spinal, epidural, leg block

Comments: This operation is typically performed on healthy, young, athletic types, who don't present great anesthetic challenges. The choice of anesthetic is typically a matter of preference on the part of the surgeon and patient, rather than a medical necessity.

A tourniquet is typically used to minimize bleeding into the joint space. (See the discussion of tourniquet considerations at the beginning of this chapter.) Since tourniquet time should be limited to 2 hours, the operation shouldn't take much longer than that.

Injecting the joint space with bupivacaine and morphine at the end of the procedure will greatly minimize postoperative pain, even though there aren't supposed to be any narcotic receptors there.

Rotator Cuff Surgery

Description: The front of the shoulder is opened, various muscle layers are transgressed, and the shoulder joint is exposed. There are a variety of operations done, depending on the patient's problem, but they all mostly consist of using really big sutures to hold muscle and tendons together that have ripped apart.

Position:	Semi-Fowler's ("beach chair")
Estimated time:	3 hours
Estimated blood loss:	200 ml; type and cross-match 2 units
Need for muscle relaxation:	Required for surgical manipulation
Indicated monitors:	Standard, Foley
Postoperative analgesia:	III
Acceptable techniques:	GETA; may be combined with an interscalene block

Comments: Fortunately, it's mostly healthy young people who rip their shoulders up, so there's not usually a whole lot of coexisting disease. A hefty anesthetic is usually required, though, since shoulder surgery is enormously stimulating.

Muscle relaxation is critical to surgical exposure and repair.

Don't put any lines or monitors on the operative arm; the surgeon will be manipulating it extensively.

Tape your endotracheal tube securely in place. You won't see it again once the drapes go up.

Some shoulder surgeries can be done under regional anesthesia alone, combining an interscalene block with some local for the skin dermatomes. Your surgeon needs to be quick and efficient, however, and your patient needs to be especially cooperative.

An interscalene block combined with a general anesthetic will provide excellent intraoperative stability and postoperative pain relief, but be aware that the surgery itself can injure the brachial plexus. If the patient has a new neurologic deficit postoperatively, it may be impossible to determine if it was caused by the surgery or the anesthesia, but you can probably guess who the surgeon will blame.

Tendon Repair (Hand)

Description: The surgeon opens the skin over the severed tendons (if there's not already a big hole there), fishes around for the severed ends, and reattaches them.

Position:	Supine
Estimated time:	1 hour
Estimated blood loss:	Minimal
Need for muscle relaxation:	Very helpful for the surgeon
Indicated monitors:	Standard
Postoperative analgesia:	II
Acceptable techniques:	GA, arm block, Bier block, local

Comments: Don't put any monitors or IVs on the affected side.

Plan on the surgeon using a tourniquet.

Expect a fairly long closure, including a complicated dressing and splint.

Carpal Tunnel Release

Description: The surgeon makes a zig-zagging incision on the anterior wrist, explores the carpal tunnel, and releases the retinaculum that is compressing the space.

Position:	Supine
Estimated time:	1 hour
Estimated blood loss:	Minimal
Need for muscle relaxation:	None
Indicated monitors:	Standard
Postoperative analgesia:	II
Acceptable techniques:	GA, arm block, Bier block, local

Comments: The choice of anesthetic is a matter for discussion among you, the patient, and the surgeon. This is about as short and peripheral an operation as you can get, and almost any approach will be reasonable. Make sure your surgeon can do the case in less than 90 minutes if you are contemplating a Bier block.

Don't plan on using the operative arm for IVs or monitors; the surgeon will need it for the tourniquet.

If you are going to use a regional anesthetic, make sure you have thoroughly documented the patient's neurologic status first!

Digit Reimplantation

Description: Severed digits are reattached, including microscopic repairs of the involved nerves, arteries, and veins, and macro repairs of the tendons, muscles, and skin.

Position:	Supine
Estimated time:	4 hours per digit
Estimated blood loss:	Minimal, but type and crossmatch 2 units anyway
Need for muscle relaxation:	Required
Indicated monitors:	Standard, Foley
Postoperative analgesia:	II
Acceptable techniques:	Regional, GETA

Comments: Typically these patients are young and healthy, with no associated injuries.

Plan on a rapid-sequence induction. Put your monitors (and your IV) on the other arm.

Although you may start with a regional technique, you will almost always end up with a general anesthetic a few hours later. Regional sympathectomy is good for blood flow in the repaired vessels, though.

Good muscle relaxation is required for the more delicate portions of the surgery.

A tourniquet will typically be placed and will be used intermittently throughout the surgery.

Maintaining the patient's temperature at or above normal is a good way to keep perfusion up and is usually not too difficult if the hand is the only part of the patient exposed. Keeping the blood volume and hematocrit up are also good ideas.

Maintaining vigilance may become a problem as the case drags on. If you get bored, ask the surgeon to tell you about the use of leeches postoperatively to reduce swelling in the reimplanted digit.

Total Knee Replacement

Description: The knee joint is opened from the front and the femoral and tibial ends are reshaped (using a power saw) into supports for the new metallic joint, which is then pounded and (possibly) cemented into either side. Postoperatively, the knee is kept from scarring down by use of a continuous passive motion (CPM) machine to maintain muscle strength and joint flexibility.

Position:	Supine
Estimated time:	4 hours
Estimated blood loss:	500 ml; type and cross-match 2 units
Need for muscle relaxation:	Helpful for surgical manipulation
Indicated monitors:	Standard, Foley; consider A-line
Postoperative analgesia:	IV, due to the CPM machine
Acceptable techniques:	GETA, epidural, spinal, or combined

Comments: The patient may be old and osteoarthritic, with other medical problems, or young and unlucky in his or her choice of athletic activity.

Epidural anesthesia is probably the best choice here, because of its ability to carry into the postoperative period. CPM is incredibly painful otherwise.

As with any total joint surgery, strict adherence to sterile technique is required. Infection of a metallic joint may well lead to amputation of the limb or complete fusion of the joint.

Although methylmethacrylate cement is often used to secure the prosthesis, hemodynamic complications are rare. This is because a tourniquet is typically used for the case and blocks the systemic uptake of the cement toxins (preventing the circulation of the methylmethacrylate monomer).

Total Hip Replacement

Description: The hip is opened via a long lateral incision, the greater trochanter is detached, the head and neck of the femur are removed, the acetabulum is ground out, and a metal ball and socket are installed. The socket is held in place with screws and sometimes with cement. The femoral component is pounded down the shaft of the femur, sometimes with cement. The greater trochanter is replaced, and the incision is closed.

Position:	Lateral decubitus
Estimated time:	5 hours
Estimated blood loss:	700 ml, type and cross-match 4 units
Need for muscle relaxation:	Helpful for exposure and manipulation
Indicated monitors:	Standard, Foley, A-line; consider CVP/PA
Postoperative analgesia:	III
Acceptable techniques:	GETA, epidural, or combined

Comments: The patients are usually old and may be somewhat debilitated. Young patients present for this operation with juvenile rheumatoid arthritis (which will impact your anesthetic in many other ways) or avascular necrosis secondary to steroid use. If the latter, make sure that they get their stress-dose steroids.

Hip surgery can be protracted and bloody, so close attention to fluid management and patient warming is essential. Have an abundance of IV access, and follow the hematocrit closely.

Methylmethacrylate cement can cause impressive hypotension, as can embolism of fat or marrow from the femur. It is imperative to have the patient's tank full before the surgeon picks up the hammer and starts pounding on the femoral component.

Misplaced acetabular screws can hit the iliac artery or its branches on the inside of the pelvis. This causes impressive retroperitoneal bleeding that may not be apparent on the surgical side of the bone. Maintain a high index of suspicion for this problem.

Epidural anesthesia has been shown to reduce overall blood loss and lead to a lower incidence of deep venous thrombosis (DVT) than general anesthesia. It is not known whether this effect applies to combined anesthetics or not, although the presumption is that it probably does. An epidural infusion may be good for the short term postoperatively but only for the first 24 hours. After that most patients will be taking PO and will be mobile.

On the down side, the patient will be receiving DVT prophylaxis and may even have gotten a dose of crystalline warfarin sodium (Coumadin) before coming to the OR. We generally feel that the benefit of an epidural outweighs the risk of its placement in a mildly anticoagulated patient, but this may vary from situation to situation.

Strict sterile technique is essential for any total joint replacement.

Total Shoulder Replacement

Description: The shoulder joint is opened, the socket is reamed, the humeral head is removed, and both sides of the joint are replaced with metal. Screws hold the socket in place, while a shaft extending down the humerus holds the ball. Cement may be used to secure the components.

Position:	Semi-Fowler's ("beach chair")
Estimated time:	5 hours
Estimated blood loss:	300 ml; type and cross-match 2 units
Need for muscle relaxation:	Required for surgical manipulation
Indicated monitors:	Standard, Foley; consider an A-line
Postoperative analgesia:	III
Acceptable techniques:	GETA; may combine with an interscalene block

Comments: This operation is relatively new and is still being done mostly on healthy patients. It's not the blood-bath that a hip replacement is, but many of the same concerns apply.

Don't put any IV lines or monitors on the operative extremity or in the ipsilateral neck.

Be wary of methylmethacrylate-induced hypotension. Tank the patient up before the cement goes in and you'll usually avoid any great dip in blood pressure. Reaming the humerus and pounding in the humeral component are usually well tolerated, and you probably don't need to place a central venous pressure monitor.

This operation can take a long time, especially if your surgeon is just learning it. Pay attention to the patient's temperature, be aware of total blood loss (mostly oozing from cut bone), and allow plenty of time for your anesthetic to wear off at the end.

You won't have very good access to the airway once the surgery commences, so make sure that the endotracheal tube is adequately secured.

An interscalene block can be a nice adjuvant for your general anesthetic and will provide an excellent start to your postoperative analgesia. The surgery itself can cause injury to the nerves in the brachial plexus that may be indistinguishable postoperatively from injury caused by the regional anesthetic. Your best policy is to warn the patient of this ahead of time and avoid regional procedures in very skittish patients.

Although not common, air embolization can occur through open sinuses in the bone. Maintain a high index of suspicion for this problem.

Laminectomy/Discectomy

Description: The surgeon makes a vertical midline incision in the back and separates the muscle layers down to the spine. Various power tools are used to take off one or more laminae, decompressing the spinal canal and providing the surgeon access to the protruding portions of intervertebral disc, which are then ripped out with something from Dad's toolbox. Depending on how much instability has been created, a bone graft may be placed between the laminae, using either banked bone or a fresh piece nibbled off the iliac crest. Closure is usually fairly rapid.

Position:	Prone on one of several frames; rarely kneeling
Estimated time:	2 hours
Estimated blood loss:	200 ml, type and cross-match 2 units
Need for muscle relaxation:	Helpful
Indicated monitors:	Standard
Postoperative analgesia:	II
Acceptable techniques:	GETA

Comments: Back surgery patients are usually fairly healthy otherwise but may have been playing the chronic pain game for a long time. Make sure they get their regular analgesics (excepting nonsteroidal anti-inflammatory drugs [NSAIDs]) up to the time of surgery, and plan on a very gradual taper postoperatively. Local anesthetics injected into the wound during closure will help with postop analgesia.

The anesthesia usually begins supine, on a stretcher, and the patient is then turned prone onto the operating table. This is a good time for IVs to come out and monitors to be lost, so pay close attention. The arms are either tucked at the sides or extended out and forward (the "Superman position"). In the latter case your antecubital IV will probably stop working, so don't put it there in the first place.

An operation in the prone position means that you will want to secure your endotracheal tube very carefully. Be wary of your tape loosening as saliva soaks through it.

You will also want to check the patient's positioning before letting the surgeon start the prep. Make sure that the face, ears, arms, breasts, genitals, and legs are all comfortably arranged, and that all of your IV lines and monitors are still working.

Document all pre-existing neurologic deficits carefully.

Muscle relaxation is very reassuring for you, the anesthetist, because it reduces the chance that the patient will cough and buck and lose the endotracheal tube. The lack of relaxation is comforting for the surgeons, because they can count on something twitching if they hit a nerve root. We usually try to keep the patient titrated to about one twitch on a train of four, which we hope will satisfy everyone.

Anesthetic alternatives include doing the case with a spinal or epidural (allowing the surgeon to provide a top-up dose if needed) or intubating the patient awake, nasally, and allowing the patient to position himself or herself on the table before inducing general anesthesia. A nasal intubation will secure the tube better than an oral approach. Both options help avoid some of the dangers of turning and positioning a patient under general anesthesia, but both will require careful preplanning and discussion with the patient and surgeon.

Don't wake the patient until you have turned him or her supine and checked all your monitors. Attempting to reintubate the patient in the prone position can be quite challenging. Be wary of sudden blood pressure shifts with any change in position.

Spinal Fusion

Description: The surgeon makes a long vertical midline incision over the scoliotic region of the spine, exposes all of the laminae on both sides, fastens hardware to various points above, below, and throughout the curve, and then puts in a couple of vertical rods to straighten everything out.

Position:	Prone
Estimated time:	8 hours
Estimated blood loss:	1,000 ml plus; type and crossmatch 6 units
Need for muscle relaxation:	Helpful
Indicated monitors:	Standard, Foley, A-line, somatosensory evoked potential (SSEP); consider CVP/PA lines
Postoperative analgesia:	III
Acceptable techniques:	GETA

Comments: This case is a real lulu! Expect a lot of bleeding, a lot of heat loss, and a big third-space fluid loss. Plan to have plenty of IV access, and keep the patient warm from the start.

Associated disease states with scoliosis include restrictive lung disease, malignant hyperthermia, airway anomalies, neurologic deficits, and neuromuscular diseases such as muscular dystrophy.

For any surgery in the prone position, make sure your endotracheal tube is well secured and that all the patient's pressure points are well padded. If the arms are tucked at the sides, make sure that all your lines and monitors are working before allowing the surgeon to start prepping, and don't put the IV in the antecubital fossa in the first place.

One of the big questions with scoliosis surgery is whether the surgeon has distracted (straightened) the spinal cord enough or too much. There are two common approaches for assessing neurologic function intraop: SSEPs and the wake-up test.

SSEPs measure the brainstem response to a stimulus provided at a distal sensory nerve, typically the posterior tibial. If the spinal cord gets stretched and ischemic the SSEP signal will change (typically decreased amplitude and increased latency) and you will be able to tell the surgeon that a problem exists. Setting up and interpreting an SSEP requires a well-trained technician.

The wake-up test is just that and is intended to measure motor function. It is therefore complementary to the SSEP, rather than redundant, and you may be asked to do both. When the surgeon has finished straightening out the cord, you will be asked to awaken the patient enough to find out if the toes still wiggle on command. There are a lot of anesthetic recipes available for doing this, but we like an approach involving a narcotic infusion, a minimum of volatile anesthetic, and a relaxant. When wake-up time approaches, the volatile anesthetic (ideally, desflurane) is turned off, the relaxant (ideally mivacurium) is allowed to resolve, and the patient is interrogated. With luck (and the right dose of narcotics) the patient will follow the commands you give, without a whole lot of unsightly coughing or bucking. It's a good idea to warn the patient about the test before starting the case, since they have a fair chance of remembering it later. It's also a good idea not to use neuromuscular reversal agents or naloxone, since you are going to want to put the patient immediately back to sleep.

Urology

Surgery on the male (and occasionally female) reproductive and urinary tracts spans the full range from minor procedures done with local anesthesia and sedation (vasectomies) to full-blown day-long dog-and-pony shows involving every monitor invented, the entire contents of your blood bank, and a broad range of vasoactive substances. This is one of the reasons we've always enjoyed urology. (Another reason is that almost all of the urologists we've met have been nice people and good surgeons.) Also, for many of us, the cystoscopy room represents our start in anesthesia and our earliest experience with mask cases and spinal blocks.

In general, urology divides into closed cases and open cases. The former group usually involves surgery through a cystoscope and is characterized by brevity, rapid finishes, and no postoperative pain. These are the cases for mask general anesthesia or short-acting spinals. They used to be boring to watch, but the advent of quality video equipment and indirect surgical techniques has made them much more entertaining.

The open cases usually involve surgery on the kidneys, bladder, or prostate and may include substantial blood loss and impressive postoperative pain. These cases do well with combined epidural and general anesthetics, or with more obscure techniques like spinal catheters (a good save when you wet tap the patient).

Urology patients, in general, tend to be sicker than average. The typical prostate surgery patient, either for a transurethral resection of prostate (TURP) or an open resection, is 65 years old, hypertensive, and a smoker, with a history of angina and chronic obstructive pulmonary disease (COPD). Fortunately, they are usually happy to have regional anesthesia and are cooperative and pleasant people. Many patients with bladder tumors have had dozens of cystoscopies and could probably put their own spinals in if you gave them a good mirror. These patients will usually have a very good idea of what they like and don't like in an anesthetic and will be happy to tell you, if you're smart enough to ask.

Circumcision

Description: "Just a little bit off the top, please." The surgeon pulls up the foreskin, cuts it off short, and sutures the loose edges together.

Position:	Supine
Estimated time:	30 minutes
Estimated blood loss:	Minimal
Need for muscle relaxation:	None
Indicated monitors:	Standard
Postoperative analgesia:	II; penile block by surgeons, caudal, PO medications
Acceptable techniques:	GA; local for adults and newborns

Comments: This procedure can usually be done with a mask general anesthetic, especially if your surgeon is swift. If the airway gets ugly, you can always intubate in the middle of the procedure. The surgeon is usually far enough away that you won't interfere with things.

A penile block by the surgeon at the end of the case is usually all the postoperative analgesia you need, although you may also choose to do a caudal block. If the child seems cranky postop anyway, consider the psychosocial issues involved and refer him to a good Freudian psychiatrist.

Hypospadias Repair

Description: Typically performed in children, this operation is done to correct abnormalities in the terminal urethra and involves creating a conduit for urine that reaches all the way to the distal meatus.

Position:	Supine
Estimated time:	2–3 hours
Estimated blood loss:	Minimal
Need for muscle relaxation:	None
Indicated monitors:	Standard
Postoperative analgesia:	II; PO medications, caudal or penile block
Acceptable techniques:	General, combined caudal and general

Comments: All of the usual pediatric concerns apply. The patient can be anywhere from a few months to a few years old.

There are usually no associated abnormalities accompanying hypospadias.

The length of surgery is related to the severity of the defect.

No Foley is available for monitoring urine output.

Older kids will have psychosocial issues associated with genital surgery. This may cause increased regressive behavior and preoperative separation anxiety.

Orchiopexy

Description: The surgeon makes an incision in the inguinal crease (as for a hernia), pulls down an improperly descended testicle, stuffs it into the scrotum, and tacks it down there.

Position:	Supine
Estimated time:	30–60 minutes
Estimated blood loss:	Minimal
Need for muscle relaxation:	May be necessary, especially in children
Indicated monitors:	Standard
Postoperative analgesia:	II; PO analgesics, caudal block in kids
Acceptable techniques:	General, spinal in adults (T-6 level)

Comments: Traction on the testicular apparatus can be quite stimulating and requires a fairly high level of block.

Vagal responses (hypotension and bradycardia) can occur with testicular manipulation.

Postoperative emesis is quite common. Aggressive treatment with droperidol or metoclopramide is probably indicated.

Penile Prosthesis

Description: The penis is opened lengthwise or at its base and one of several varieties of hardware is inserted. High-tech pump model prostheses also require a scrotal incision.

Position:	Supine
Estimated time:	90–180 minutes
Estimated blood loss:	Minimal
Need for muscle relaxation:	None
Indicated monitors:	Standard
Postoperative analgesia:	II; PO medications
Acceptable techniques:	GETA, spinal, epidural (T-12 level)

Comments: The patient is usually healthy, and boredom is probably your biggest anesthetic concern.

Many patients desire general anesthesia for social reasons; if the patient does remain awake, you should maintain an appropriate sense of decorum.

Cystoscopy

Description: A cystoscope is inserted via the urethra into the bladder, which is kept distended by a continuous flow of irrigating solution. Sometimes all that's required is a look around, but biopsies of the prostate or bladder are often performed. Bladder tumors may be resected this way, using an electrocautery device.

Position:	Lithotomy
Estimated time:	15–60 minutes
Estimated blood loss:	Minimal
Need for muscle relaxation:	None
Indicated monitors:	Standard
Postoperative analgesia:	I; None
Acceptable techniques:	General, spinal, or epidural (T-10 level)

Comments: In females a simple cystoscopy can be easily accomplished with just local anesthesia. Males usually require something more. Local anesthetic instilled into the bladder will sometimes suffice.

This procedure ends abruptly. Good communication is essential to avoid overanesthetizing.

IV methylene blue or indigo carmine may be requested by the surgeon to help view the ureteral openings in the bladder. Either of these agents can cause erroneously low pulse oximeter readings when given IV. Wear gloves when drawing the dye up to avoid staining your fingers.

Keeping the spinal level low (around T-10) will allow you to recognize the typical pain in the belly and shoulder that is associated with bladder perforation.

Percutaneous Nephrostomy (PCN) Tube Placement

Description: A collection of pus in the renal pelvis is aspirated percutaneously, under ultrasound guidance, and a drainage tube is then placed through the same tract.

Position:	Prone
Estimated time:	1 hour
Estimated blood loss:	Minimal
Need for muscle relaxation:	None
Indicated monitors:	Standard
Postoperative analgesia:	II; PO medications
Acceptable techniques:	Epidural, spinal, MAC, or GETA

Comments: Because of the awkward position, regional anesthesia is usually easier and quicker than a general.

This procedure can be done with just local anesthesia, but it is usually fairly painful.

Fluoroscopy with contrast material may be part of the procedure. Watch for anaphylaxis and have your epinephrine ready.

This procedure often precedes, by a day or two, a more definitive procedure to address the infected, obstructed kidney. Epidurals and monitoring lines placed for the tube placement can be left in place for the bigger operation to follow.

Ureteral Stone Removal
(Via Cystoscope)

Description: A cystoscope is inserted via the urethra into the bladder, which is distended by a continuous flow of an irrigating solution. A fiberoptic scope is then threaded up the appropriate ureter and the offending kidney stone addressed. Sometimes it can simply be grabbed and dragged out. Other times it is broken up by a laser or ultrasonic probe and the pieces are grabbed or flushed out.

Position:	Lithotomy
Estimated time:	1–6 hours (truly indeterminate)
Estimated blood loss:	Minimal
Need for muscle relaxation:	Yes. Patient must hold still!
Indicated monitors:	Standard
Postoperative analgesia:	III; may have significant renal colic postop
Acceptable techniques:	GETA, spinal, or epidural (T-4 level)

Comments: The high regional level indicated is because of the need to anesthetize the renal pelvis, which can be significantly stimulated during the procedure.

This procedure may end abruptly! Stone basketing or demolition can be very tricky, and there's no way to tell ahead of time how long things are going to take. Once the stone is removed, however, the operation is over; there's no closure time to allow you to plan your wake-up.

Frequent x-rays or repeated fluoroscopy are common.

Inadvertent perforation of the ureter is a bad complication. You should avoid any patient movement, if possible.

Lithotripsy

Description: An ultrasonic wave generator is focused through the skin on a kidney stone, under fluoroscopic guidance, and is fired several hundred times. The stone breaks into small pieces and is flushed out of the renal pelvis.

Position:	Supine or semi-Fowler's
Estimated time:	1 hour
Estimated blood loss:	None
Need for muscle relaxation:	None
Indicated monitors:	Standard; waterproof ECG leads required with older lithotripsy machines
Postoperative analgesia:	II; renal colic pain, PO medications
Acceptable techniques:	Epidural, spinal, GETA, or MAC

Comments: Older lithotripsy machines require the patient to be immersed in a large steel bathtub, raising an interesting set of issues for the anesthetist:

1. The patient has to be anesthetized and then moved into this position.
2. Immersion can cause vasodilatation and vagal responses.
3. Monitoring can be difficult. Waterproof tape is needed over the ECG pads. The arms are usually supported outside the tub. Watch for brachial plexus injuries.
4. Real anesthesia is needed with this technology (not MAC).

Newer lithotripsy machines allow the patient to lie supine on a water mattress and allow MACs or straight local procedures.

With either technique it is important to keep your equipment out of the path of the sound waves. The sound wave pulses are triggered by the ECG, so avoid slowing the heart rate too much or the procedure will take longer.

Frequent fluoroscopy is common.

It is not unusual to do a cystoscopy and stent placement prior to the lithotripsy, which may change the
patient's anesthetic requirements.

Lithotripsy is typically done on an outpatient basis in
otherwise healthy patients. Everyone will be expecting a
simple anesthetic, so the finger-pointing will be severe if
a complication occurs.

Transurethral Resection of Prostate (TURP)

Description: A cystoscope is inserted via the penis into the bladder, which is kept distended by a continuous infusion of a nonelectrolyte solution. The prostate is examined from the inside, and hypertrophic tissue is cored away with an electrically heated wire loop. Bleeding vessels and venous sinuses are coagulated, and a continuously irrigating Foley catheter is left in place.

Position:	Lithotomy
Estimated time:	1 hour
Estimated blood loss:	Hard to estimate intra-operatively. Type and crossmatch for 2 units.
Need for muscle relaxation:	None
Indicated monitors:	Standard; awake patient helpful
Postoperative analgesia:	None
Acceptable techniques:	Spinal preferred over GETA, epidural if cardio-vascular instability exists (T-10 level)

Comments: Most patients presenting for TURP will have additional medical problems, some quite severe. A careful preoperative assessment is important.

Absorption of water from the irrigating solution may cause acute hyponatremia, which will be first manifested by mental status changes but may progress to hypertension, seizures, intravascular hemolysis, and fatal cardiac rhythm abnormalities. Hypothermia may also occur. This constellation of symptoms is collectively known as the "TURP syndrome."

Regional anesthesia reduces the incidence of deep venous thrombosis and may help limit blood loss. Most important, regional anesthesia allows the ability to communicate with the patient, monitoring mental status for the central nervous system manifestations of TURP syndrome.

A level at T-10 will allow for the detection of pain (typ-

ically in the right shoulder) if the surgeons inadvertently perforate the prostatic capsule.

Air embolization has been reported from empty irrigation bags sucked out by negative pressure in the prostatic venous sinuses.

This operation finishes very quickly. One moment the
surgeon is cauterizing the inside of the prostatic capsule,
and the next moment everything is pulled out and you're
wondering how to get rid of 1.5% isoflurane. Another
good reason to use regional!

Close PACU monitoring of these patients is a good
idea, since they can develop electrolyte abnormalities or
obstructions of their irrigating Foley catheters.

Open Prostatectomy

Description: Through a midline abdominal incision, the peritoneum is retracted superiorly and the prostate is shelled out of its capsule and removed. The urethra-bladder connection is then repaired. Lymph nodes are sampled from the pelvic side walls and the retroperitoneum.

Position:	Supine or lithotomy
Estimated time:	3 hours
Estimated blood loss:	700 ml; type and cross-match 4 units
Need for muscle relaxation:	Required
Indicated monitors:	Standard, Foley, A-line; low threshold for CVP/PA lines
Postoperative analgesia:	III; continuous epidural, intrathecal narcotics, PCA
Acceptable techniques:	GETA; combined epidural and general is good

Comments: Epidural anesthesia reduces the incidence of DVTs and decreases surgical blood loss.

Blood loss can be impressive for the (usually) short period when the prostate is being shelled out. Once the specimen is removed hemostasis is usually easy to achieve. You will want to have good IV access in any case.

Lymph node sampling may precede the prostatectomy if a positive result means no further surgery.

When the patient is placed in the lithotomy position your epidural catheter suddenly may become difficult to inject. This effect will typically resolve once the patient is returned to the supine position.

The Foley catheter may be only intermittently available for measuring urine output.

Warmth and fluid volume may become issues if the surgery is longer or the blood loss is greater than anticipated.

Perineal Prostatectomy

Description: A horseshoe-shaped incision is made around the perineum and the prostate is removed. The urethra is then reattached to the bladder and closed over a Foley catheter.

Position:	Extreme lithotomy with Trendelenburg
Estimated time:	3 hours
Estimated blood loss:	500 ml; type and cross-match for 2 units
Need for muscle relaxation:	Helps maintain position, ventilation
Indicated monitors:	Standard, 5-lead, Foley, A-line; CVP/PA line if your surgeons run long or the patient is sick
Postoperative analgesia:	III; epidural, intrathecal narcotics, or IV PCA
Acceptable techniques:	GETA, spinal; combined epidural/general (T-6 level)

Comments: Epidural or spinal block reduces blood loss and decreases the incidence of DVTs. Caution is required when injecting anesthetics in the Trendelenburg position!

The Foley catheter will be only intermittently available as a monitor of urine output. Invasive monitoring is therefore indicated somewhat more strongly than in a case where urine output can be closely followed.

Patients are at high risk for DVTs, presumably because of the sharp bending of the legs. Nerve injuries (peroneal, femoral, sciatic) can occur as a result of the extreme lithotomy position. Muscle breakdown and significant myoglobinemia can occur in heavy patients or long procedures. Maintain adequate hydration!

This operation is commonly preceded by a pelvic lymph node dissection. Positive nodes mean no prostatectomy.

We observed a steep learning curve on this operation with our surgeons. All of our complications (excessive blood loss and nerve damage) occurred in the first few, 6-hour long procedures. Since then our average case time is closer to 90 minutes, and we have had no more problems.

Orchiectomy

Description: The top of the scrotum is opened and the testicle is removed.

Position:	Supine
Estimated time:	30–60 minutes
Estimated blood loss:	Minimal
Need for muscle relaxation:	None
Indicated monitors:	Standard
Postoperative analgesia:	II; PO analgesics
Acceptable techniques:	GETA, spinal or epidural (T-6 level)

Comments: A high level is needed to block sensation from traction on the spermatic cord. An insufficient level will lead to nausea, restlessness, hypotension/bradycardia (vagal response), and possibly outright pain.

If the operation is being performed for testicular cancer, it may include a more extensive dissection, including retroperitoneal lymph node sampling.

If the operation is being performed for prostate cancer it will usually be a bilateral procedure, and the patient will likely be older and sicker.

A fair amount of anxiety is associated with this operation. This will be even more exacerbated if the operation is performed for a malignancy. Be generous with your preoperative anxiolysis and intraoperative sedation for regional cases.

Reimplantation of Ureters

Description: This operation is performed, usually in pediatric patients, to fix reflux at the ureteral pelvic junction. The abdomen is opened through a midline incision, and the peritoneum and its contents are retracted superiorly. The ureters are identified and dissected free, cut at the bladder end, and then reattached in a reflux-proof fashion. Stents may be placed intraoperatively, and are often left in place postoperatively.

Position:	Supine
Estimated time:	2–4 hours
Estimated blood loss:	100 ml; type and screen
Need for muscle relaxation:	Yes, for abdominal exposure
Indicated monitors:	Standard, Foley
Postoperative analgesia:	III; caudal or epidural, PCA if old enough
Acceptable techniques:	GETA, combined caudal and general

Comments: The usual pediatric considerations apply; patients can be of any age, but are most commonly 2–5 years old. Ureteral reflux is not associated with any specific congenital syndromes, but a careful look for congenital anomalies is always a good idea.

Urine output will be interrupted during the case but is a source of great concern to the urologists once their anastomoses are complete.

Pay attention to keeping the patient warm, especially if he or she is very young!

Nephrectomy

Description: A long transverse flank incision is made, the kidney is shelled out of its perinephric fat, and the ureter, artery, and vein (in that order) are identified and ligated, allowing the specimen to be removed.

Position:	Lateral, with the bed sharply flexed and in a little Trendelenburg (enough to level the surgical field). Arms are extended in front
Estimated time:	3 hours; longer for cancer surgery
Estimated blood loss:	500 ml; type and crossmatch 4 units. More for cancer surgery
Need for muscle relaxation:	Required
Indicated monitors:	Standard, Foley, A-line, 5-lead; low threshold for CVP/PA line
Postoperative analgesia:	IV
Acceptable techniques:	GETA or combined epidural and GETA (T-2 level). Be cautious with the sympathectomy in high blood loss cases.

Comments: This operation may be for benign (obstructing stones, pyelonephritis, nonfunctioning, living related donation) or malignant (renal cell carcinoma [CA], transitional cell CA, Wilms' tumor) causes. Benign operations are usually very straightforward. Malignant operations may involve extensive additional dissection to allow en bloc resection of the kidney and everything around it. Dissecting through a renal tumor makes an impressively bloody mess. And some tumors have the nasty habit of spreading locally into the venous system (up the vena cava) or down the ureter. We know of one nephrectomy for renal cell CA where cardiac bypass was requested to allow resection of tumor that had extended all the way into the right atrium!

Deliberate or inadvertent violation of the diaphragm is common. Unexplained hypotension and increasing airway pressures could mean a pneumothorax.

Urine output is usually not a problem if the other kidney is functioning adequately, but this is something you should pay close attention to.

Be prepared to deal with very rapid bleeding. It is not uncommon for an accessory renal vein to be discovered as it rips off the vena cava when the specimen is being removed. Dose your epidural with appropriate caution early in the case, using either short-acting local anesthetics or narcotics alone.

Keep the patient warm from the start.

Cystectomy/Ileal Loop

Description: Through a long abdominal incision, the bladder is dissected out and removed. The ureters are then anastomosed to a short section of small intestine (removed from continuity with the rest of the bowel), which is brought out to the surface as an enterostomy.

Position:	Supine
Estimated time:	6 hours
Estimated blood loss:	1,000 ml; type and cross-match 4 units
Need for muscle relaxation:	Yes, for surgical exposure
Indicated monitors:	Standard, A-line; low threshold for CVP/PA lines
Postoperative analgesia:	IV; epidural infusion or PCA
Acceptable techniques:	GETA or combined

Comments: This is a big case! Dissection can be tedious if adhesions exist or if an en bloc cancer specimen is desired.

Attention to warming is important.

Substantial fluid shifts can occur, and there is no way to monitor urine output for most of the case. The patient has usually been bowel prepped and will typically arrive in the OR already dehydrated. Get yourself plenty of IV access before starting.

Cancer cases can lead to a lot of blood loss.

Oral Surgery

"Open wide...."

Oral surgery is a small niche, but it carries a certain potential for excitement. The patients are usually young and usually healthy, and the procedures are usually completely elective. Postponing cases is not uncommon. If you were going to have your jaw wired shut for 3 weeks, you wouldn't want to start out with a cold.

Jaw wiring will follow any case designed to improve the patient's occlusion, the match made by the upper and lower teeth. Jaw wiring implies a nasal intubation, and it demands extreme caution before extubating. The airway must be thoroughly suctioned, the throat pack removed, the patient wide awake, and equipment on hand to quickly cut the wires, if necessary. Doing so will potentially destroy the surgical repair, but given a choice between breathing and having straight teeth, most patients will opt for the former.

During the operation, after your nasal intubation and before you start worrying about the extubation, you will have very little contact with the airway. Oral surgeons get more anesthesia training than most surgeons, and one of the reasons is that they spend a lot of time messing around with the proximal airway. (The other reason, by the way, is that they give a lot of their own anesthesia in the clinic or private office and have to have some basic understanding of monitored care and airway management.) Once your tube goes in, the surgeon will descend on the oral cavity like a vulture, resecuring your tube, packing the throat, and wielding fists full of sharp instruments.

Postoperatively the patients are often impressively swollen, despite controlled hypotension intraop, limited fluid administration, and the liberal use of dexamethasone. Taking them intubated to the PACU and sitting them up for a while before extubating is often the better part of valor.

What will you get out of working on the oral surgery service? Some nasal intubations, the occasional arterial line and hypotensive technique, and some scary extubations. Enjoy!

Dental Extractions (Odontectomy)

Description: The oral surgeon opens the patient's mouth and pulls out the offending teeth. Drilling may occasionally be necessary to free up teeth that are buried or stuck.

Position:	Supine or semi-sitting, mouth open
Estimated time:	60 minutes
Estimated blood loss:	Minimal
Need for muscle relaxation:	Helpful
Indicated monitors:	Standard
Postoperative analgesia:	II
Acceptable techniques:	GETA, local

Comments: Most people having teeth pulled are healthy adolescents or young adults; unfortunately for you, most of these patients will have local anesthesia only, far from your OR. The patients you see will either have severely impacted teeth, which are hard to remove, or will be mentally retarded, chronically ill, or just plain uncooperative. Still, if it wasn't a difficult job, they wouldn't need someone as good as you to do it.

The oral surgeon will prefer you to intubate the patient nasally, so that neither of you has to worry about dislodging the tube during the procedure. The normal pattern is to topicalize patients either before they go to sleep or just after, when you're waiting for the muscle relaxant to hit. Consider lidocaine jelly and phenylephrine hydrochloride (Neo-Synephrine) on a nasal trumpet as an easy way to do this.

After you have induced anesthesia and topicalized the nose, you can pass the endotracheal tube into the back of the throat, look around with the laryngoscope, and then either advance the tube directly through the cords or use a pair of McGill forceps to help guide it.

Use a tube that's a size smaller than normal. Placing the tube in a bottle of sterile saline in the blanket warmer for an hour or so before induction will soften it up, making it less likely to cause a nosebleed when you use it. On the other hand, this technique will also soften the natural curve of the tube and make it more likely that you will need the McGill's to place it.

The surgeon will place a throat pack before pulling the teeth. Make sure this is out at the end of the case and make sure you have thoroughly suctioned the patient's pharynx and stomach before extubating. Even a little blood in the vicinity of the vocal cords can cause laryngospasm. The oral surgeon will typically want to be around when the patient is extubated.

The best way to manage postop pain is to have the surgeon inject some local anesthetic before extracting the teeth, just as if there were no general anesthesia involved.

Bilateral Split Sagittal Osteotomy (BSSO)

Description: The purpose of this procedure is to length-en and change the angle of the mandible to bring the lower teeth into better alignment with the upper teeth. An incision is made on each side of the oral cavity, and the mandible is exposed. The bone is cut through with a saw, then shifted to its new position and secured with plates and screws. Bone autograft from the hip may be used to fill in any bony defects. The jaw is wired shut at the end of the case.

Position:	Semi-Fowler's
Estimated time:	3 hours
Estimated blood loss:	400 ml; type and cross-match 2 units
Need for muscle relaxation:	Helpful
Indicated monitors:	Standard, Foley; A-line for deliberate hypotension
Postoperative analgesia:	III
Acceptable techniques:	GETA

Comments: The patient is usually healthy and eager for the operation.

Nasal intubation is required, both to keep the tube out of the surgeon's way and because the jaw will be wired shut before the patient is extubated. Intubation can usu-ally be accomplished with the patient asleep, using the McGill forceps, but you should take a good look at the airway before beginning.

This operation is frequently combined with a LeFort osteotomy (see the following section) to produce an all-day jaw wrangling. Hemodilution or deliberate hypoten-sion may be necessary to avoid having to transfuse the patient, especially if autologous bone is being harvested from the hip.

Help the surgeon make sure that the throat pack comes out before the jaw wires go in.

The patient will be quite swollen at the end of the case. Give some dexamethasone to help with this, keep him or her head-up in the PACU, and don't extubate until you feel that conditions are perfect.

When you do extubate, make sure you have a pair of wire snips on hand to allow you to open the mouth in an emergency. Laryngospasm and vomiting are two good things to avoid in this situation. Suction the patient's mouth and stomach before extubating.

LeFort Procedure

Description: Le Fort was a nineteenth-century French surgeon who achieved immortality by dropping human skulls face-first onto a concrete floor. He published a classification of the resulting maxillary fractures that has stood the test of time, applying equally well to our present generation of face-meets-windshield injuries. In the elective circumstance a LeFort procedure refers to the deliberate bilateral fracture and resetting of the maxilla (using small plates and screws) to provide better dental occlusion.

Position:	Semi-Fowler's, head up
Estimated time:	4 hours
Estimated blood loss:	500 ml; type and cross-match 2 units
Need for muscle relaxation:	Helpful
Indicated monitors:	Standard, Foley; A-line for deliberate hypotension
Postoperative analgesia:	III
Acceptable techniques:	GETA

Comments: The patients are generally healthy.

A nasal intubation is required, since the surgeon will be wiring the jaw shut at the end of the case. Most of the time the intubation can be done with the patient asleep, using the McGill forceps if necessary to get the tube in the right place. Occasionally the patient will have a bad enough overbite that you are concerned about your ability to see the cords with a laryngoscope. These patients should be intubated awake, either blindly or with a fiberoptic bronchoscope.

The LeFort procedure is very often combined with a BSSO (see the preceding section) as a way of bringing the maxilla and the mandible into proper alignment. This combined procedure can make for a long day in the OR and should make you think about techniques like deliberate hypotension or hemodilution to avoid having to transfuse a healthy patient. Hypotension can usually be achieved with high-dose isoflurane without the need for additional drugs.

The surgeon will use a throat pack to minimize blood loss into the airway. Make sure this comes out before the teeth are wired together, and document it on your record.

The upper airway will be impressively edematous at the end of the procedure. Don't be in any rush to extubate the patient. Sometimes sitting around the PACU for a while with the tube in, the head up, and the dexamethasone circulating is just the ticket. When you do extubate, make sure conditions are perfect: Suction out the patient thoroughly (including the stomach), have him or her wide awake and breathing well, and have equipment on hand to cut the jaw wires if things don't work out.

Ophthalmology

Ophthalmology is characterized by sick patients, usually at the extremes of age, having minor surgery. This is the service where you can learn how to give a really effective MAC, using midazolam, fentanyl, propofol, droperidol, tape, reassurance, and hand-holding. Patients may be any age—from premature infants to centenarians—and often have coexisting medical problems about which the surgeon is only marginally informed.

Working in your favor is the fact that fluid shifts are usually minimal, that you don't have to give a lot of anesthesia, and that the cases are almost always completely elective. You can postpone the case if things don't look right. On the other hand, the patient has to be able to lie flat and hold still for most eye cases, both difficult skills for those at the extremes of life. If you accidentally oversedate someone, your access to the airway is poor and the surgeon will be unhappy about having to stop.

General anesthetics protect the airway and keep the patient still but may run you afoul of the patient's medical disease. Waking up tends to be slow, since the pain produced by the incision is minimal (and often blocked by local anesthetics anyway).

An eye block works well for many ophthalmology cases and can be accompanied by a modest amount of sedation. The surgeon will do the block in most cases, and most of the time it will work great. Every once in a while, though, the surgeon will prove that there is a direct connection between the eye and the brain along the optic nerve and will induce the highest of spinal blocks. You will need to be prepared for this eventuality by having the patient well monitored and having resuscitation gear close at hand.

One thing to keep in mind during any eye surgery is the potential for an oculocardiac reflex. Pressure on the eye can cause a vagal response manifesting as sudden bradycardia and hypotension. A good eye block will remove the afferent arm of this reflex, and a slug of atropine will treat the efferent. Asking the surgeon to stop manipulating the eye will usually fix the acute problem, although occasionally bradycardia progresses to asystole and a minute or two of CPR may be necessary to circulate the atropine. (We hate it when that happens.)

Unfortunately for you, most of ophthalmology involves the kind of no-glory anesthesia that we've always hated. If things go well, that's great, but that's what was expected. If thing's go badly, it'll be nobody's fault but your own. Oh, well, someone has to do it.

Cataract Extraction

Description: The surgeon makes a small incision around the rim of the cornea, pops out the cataract (or melts it ultrasonically, or whatever), and stuffs in a plastic lens. The incision is closed with a few quick stitches, and the operation is over.

Position:	Supine
Estimated time:	2 hours
Estimated blood loss:	Minimal
Need for muscle relaxation:	None
Indicated monitors:	Standard
Postoperative analgesia:	I
Acceptable techniques:	MAC, local, GETA

Comments: The patient is usually in the geriatric set and may have a problem list as long as your arm. The secret when doing the preoperative assessment is to remind yourself periodically that having a cataract removed under a retrobulbar block with you in attendance is probably safer for patients than lying at home in their own beds. After all, they aren't hooked to a pulse oximeter at home. The key question to ask is, "Can you lie flat on your back for a couple of hours?" End-stage cardiac or respiratory patients may not be able to do that, which will screw things up mightily. We have occasionally persuaded our surgeon to operate standing up (rather than sitting), with the patient in a semi-Fowler's position, but this creates as many problems as it solves. The microscope may require special adjustment to focus higher up, and everybody's rhythm will be thrown off.

You would probably rather listen to the surgeon complain, though, than risk giving general anesthesia to a cardiac or respiratory cripple. We reserve the GETA option only for uncooperative patients (typically those with mild dementia) who are otherwise healthy. We ask the surgeon to put a retrobulbar block in anyway, so that we can keep the anesthesia light.

And speaking of retrobulbar blocks—the surgeon will typically do it, although it's fun to watch and learn about. A little local in the vicinity of the temple will numb the cornea and the skin below the eye and make it easy for the surgeon to pop into the retrobulbar space. We use just a little bit of propofol for this part of the procedure, with oxygen and monitors in place. Once the block is in, most patients won't need more than a little oxygen blowing under the drapes and a hand to hold. Be cautious with sedation since it's very easy to overdo it in these patients.

Surgery in the retrobulbar space can produce an oculocardiac response (hypotension and bradycardia) as well as nausea and vomiting. Be prepared for both.

Scleral Buckle

Description: It's hard to see exactly what the surgeon is doing in there, but the basic idea is to open the globe of the eye and reattach the retina to the back wall without actually traumatizing it.

Position:	Supine
Estimated time:	3 hours
Estimated blood loss:	Minimal
Need for muscle relaxation:	Not needed
Indicated monitors:	Standard
Postoperative analgesia:	II
Acceptable techniques:	GETA

Comments: The patient can be any age but is often young and anxious about going blind. Diabetics are also prone to this condition and may have had multiple operations over the years.

Your anesthetic should be generous, to avoid movement while the surgeon is operating through the microscope. You should plan on as smooth a wake-up as you can contrive since coughing and bucking with extubation will increase intraocular pressure and may screw up the repair. Narcotics are good for this purpose.

Once in a while our surgeons want to leave a gas bubble in the globe of the eye to help hold the retina in place. Depending on the density of the substance used, you may be asked to extubate the patient prone so that the bubble will remain in the correct portion of the eye. Nitrous oxide is contraindicated no matter what the bubble's density; plan to turn it off before the bubble is placed.

Blepharoplasty

Description: The surgeon resects redundant skin from above and below the eye, leaving just enough for the eyelids to close effectively.

Position:	Supine
Estimated time:	2 hours
Estimated blood loss:	Minimal
Need for muscle relaxation:	None
Indicated monitors:	Standard
Postoperative analgesia:	II
Acceptable techniques:	MAC, GETA

Comments: The patients are usually elderly but not as sick as cataract patients. This procedure is more for cosmetic purposes than for improving vision, and the surgeon usually won't suggest it in a sicker patient.

The operation will proceed under local anesthesia since an endotracheal tube will get in the surgeon's way. Make sure your monitoring is good, that the patient is receiving enough oxygen under the drapes, and that you are close enough to hold a hand if necessary.

A four-lid blepharoplasty may become tedious for all concerned. The patient can pass the time in the pleasant glow of IV benzodiazepines, but this approach is not recommended for the anesthesia provider. You'll just have to stick it out.

Don't overdo the sedation, though, since it'll be hard (and embarrassing) to access the airway in the middle of the case.

Since the trigeminal nerve will not be blocked by the superficially applied local anesthetic, you may have to watch out for oculocardiac responses triggered by pressure on the eyeball. Treat with atropine, ephedrine, or by yelling, "Hey! Stop pushing on that!"

Foreign Body Removal

Description: The surgeon takes out the foreign body and makes whatever repairs are needed to preserve the retina, close the globe, and provide a cosmetically satisfying result.

Position:	Supine
Estimated time:	1 hour plus
Estimated blood loss:	Minimal
Need for muscle relaxation:	Helpful
Indicated monitors:	Standard; consider Foley
Postoperative analgesia:	II
Acceptable techniques:	Local, MAC, GETA

Comments: Foreign bodies that don't penetrate the globe itself can often be removed in the emergency room under topical anesthesia. Those aren't the ones you're going to get to see, however. For you we have a berserk 6-year-old with a sharpened pencil coming straight out of the eyeball and an equally berserk parent.

Remember to think about other injuries associated with trauma, particularly if a motor vehicle was involved. Give aspiration prophylaxis if time and circumstances allow.

Your mission is to get the patient anesthetized in as smooth a fashion as possible while doing everything you can to keep the patient's intraocular pressure down. Succinylcholine will cause a transient rise (not blocked by precurarization) that may nonetheless be unavoidable in some circumstances. We generally prefer a high dose of a nondepolarizing relaxant, some cricoid pressure, and a relatively rapid-sequence induction. It would be nice to do a mask induction in the pediatric patient, but the geometry of the foreign body coming out of the eye and the concern with aspiration usually lead us to bite the bullet and put in an IV first. Keep the child as quiet as possible while you do this, though, since agitation will raise the intraocular pressure. If anyone gives you a hard time, remind them that the kid was also yelling and screaming before you got there!

Intraoperative strategies to lower intraocular pressure include mannitol, furosemide, and keeping the patient's head up. Consult with the surgeon on this point.

Be generous with your anesthetic and muscle relaxant. Movement during microsurgery will make your surgeon somewhat cranky. Try to extubate without a lot of coughing and bucking since that will strain the surgical repair of the globe and potentially make the surgeon *very* cranky. Narcotics, as opposed to volatile anesthetics, are usually good for this purpose.

Strabismus Surgery

Description: This operation is actually performed on the eye muscles, rather than the globe itself, and is individualized for the particular patient. Various muscles around the eyes are either tightened or released to allow the eyes to rest in a more or less parallel position.

Position:	Supine
Estimated time:	2 hours
Estimated blood loss:	Minimal
Need for muscle relaxation:	Helpful
Indicated monitors:	Standard
Postoperative analgesia:	II
Acceptable techniques:	GETA

Comments: The usual patient is a cross-eyed 3-year-old with no other medical problems. Strabismus surgery in adults is rare. Associated anomalies are uncommon, but there is some evidence linking strabismus surgery with an increased risk of malignant hyperthermia.

Inhalation inductions are the norm. Intubation is required, to get you out of the surgeon's way.

Pressing on the eyeball can produce an oculocardiac response, characterized by bradycardia and hypotension. This response can be prevented by atropine (which you may have already given, depending on the age of the child) and treated by asking the surgeon to stop the stimulus for a minute.

Keep the anesthetic deep enough to prevent movement while the surgeon is working.

Pay attention to where the surgeon is resting his or her hands. Every so often your endotracheal tube will become mysteriously kinked....

Some prophylaxis against nausea and vomiting (droperidol and/or metoclopramide) is a good idea. The child will probably be seeing double on emergence and will have every excuse to barf all over you. Droperidol (75 µg/kg) is effective but sedating. Metoclopramide (150 µg/kg) may also be useful.

Nasolacrimal Duct Probe

Description: Following induction of anesthesia, the surgeon uses a probe to explore the nasolacrimal duct. Sometimes this is all that is required to restore its patency; other times a longer procedure is required to open it up and restore it to function.

Position:	Supine
Estimated time:	10 minutes plus
Estimated blood loss:	Minimal
Need for muscle relaxation:	None
Indicated monitors:	Standard
Postoperative analgesia:	II
Acceptable techniques:	GETA

Comments: The patient is usually a preschool child with gummy eyes but no other significant medical problems. This surgery is always elective.

If the operation is short, and your surgeon is cooperative, you can do it with a mask anesthetic alone, without starting an IV. You may have to remove the mask for a few seconds at a time to let the surgeon work, but the patient will tolerate this well if he or she is breathing spontaneously and is deeply anesthetized.

If the operation takes any time more than a few seconds we usually prefer to start an IV and intubate the child.

Inadvertent surgical pressure on the eye can produce an oculocardiac reflex. Pressure on the endotracheal tube can cause an obstruction. Don't stop paying attention!

Fluoroscein, a fluorescent yellow dye, is sometimes used to demonstrate duct patency. Make sure you suction this out carefully, since it can be a potent stimulus for laryngospasm.

Plastic Surgery

On the plastic surgery service you will mostly learn patience. The operations are slow and—well, meticulous. The patients are young and healthy, and the surgeons are not always good conversationalists.

Most of your plastic surgery time will be with healthy young people who desire an aesthetic enhancement. Since they are coming to the surgeon (and by extension, you) on a purely elective basis, they tend to approach the whole OR process more as discriminating consumers than as victims in need. This is a good service for honing your skills in interpersonal communication, gentle anxiolysis, and patient-friendly anesthesia.

Every so often, of course, a plastic surgery case will give you the opportunity to help someone who has been dealt a bad hand. Plastic surgeons may care for burn patients who often require multiple procedures over time, or they may take on interesting congenital anomalies such as cleft palates or deforming birthmarks. They also do immediate reconstructive surgery on patients who have had large cancer resections of the breast, face, or neck. These are the patients who truly merit all the compassion you can generate, as well as all your anesthetic skill.

So remember, as you watch the surgeon taking an hour and a half to close a 4-inch breast reduction incision: both of you are training for better things!

Rhinoplasty

Description: The surgeon resects part of the nasal cartilage (from the inside) to make a big nose smaller or to correct a deviated septum.

Position:	Semi-Fowler's
Estimated time:	60 minutes
Estimated blood loss:	Minimal
Need for muscle relaxation:	None
Indicated monitors:	Standard
Postoperative analgesia:	II
Acceptable techniques:	Local, MAC, GETA

Comments: Healthy patients.

This procedure is often done while the patient is under local anesthesia alone. The fact that you have been assigned to a rhinoplasty means that either the surgery or the patient is more difficult than the norm.

Even if the patient is under general anesthesia, the surgeon will probably still give some local and/or topical anesthetics to reduce intraoperative bleeding. Don't use a lot of fixed agents for this case, because the patient will have no pain at the end and may not want to wake up.

Consult with the surgeon before taping in your endotracheal tube. Tape on the face and a lot of junk in the mouth (like the oral airway bite-block) can distort the facial anatomy and screw up the surgical procedure.

Be wary of the throat pack! What goes in, must come out, at least if you want the patient to breathe after extubation. Make sure you suction the airway thoroughly to avoid laryngospasm.

Augmentation or Reduction Mammoplasty

Description: The surgeon makes a bilateral incision at the lower border of the breast and either removes some of what's there or adds some new stuff (typically a saline-filled implant).

Position:	Supine
Estimated time:	3 hours
Estimated blood loss:	300 ml; type and cross-match 2 units
Need for muscle relaxation:	None
Indicated monitors:	Standard, consider Foley
Postoperative analgesia:	II
Acceptable techniques:	GETA

Comments: The patient is usually a young healthy woman with a discrepancy between what nature supplied and what she believes to be aesthetically appropriate. This case is totally elective.

Patients with large breasts may be hard to intubate (use the short handle from obstetrics) and hard to ventilate. You may need to tolerate higher peak airway pressures than normal to keep the lungs inflated.

The surgeon will want to get to the patient before the IV starts to mark up her skin with a purple pen.

Blood loss is usually greater in a reduction mammoplasty and may be quite vigorous for a few short minutes.

Closure takes forever and is followed by an elaborate breast-binding ritual that may take up to 20 minutes. Don't wake up the patient too soon.

Breast Reconstruction

Description: The surgeon creates a new breast for the patient to replace one that has been lost to cancer. The new breast may consist of a saline-filled implant (silicone now having been banned) or a rotation flap of muscle from the abdominal wall. Reconstruction can be immediate, as part of a mastectomy, or months to years later.

Position:	Supine
Estimated time:	2 hours
Estimated blood loss:	200 ml; type and screen
Need for muscle relaxation:	None
Indicated monitors:	Standard
Postoperative analgesia:	II
Acceptable techniques:	GETA

Comments: If a reconstruction is being undertaken weeks after the resection, it usually means the patient is in remission from the cancer, so the psychiatric overlay is a bit different from the original procedure. The patient may have had radiation or chemotherapy in the interval, though, which could affect your anesthetic.

The ipsilateral arm will be off-limits for IV and blood pressure because of interruption of its lymphatic drainage during the cancer operation.

Because silicone implants have fallen into disfavor, a reconstruction nowadays may include the removal of a pre-existing implant. If the old implant has ruptured, it may be badly scarred into the surrounding tissue. Expect an implant replacement operation to be substantially longer and bloodier than a primary reconstruction.

Because aesthetics are important in this procedure, the surgeon will want a few minutes alone with the patient before the operation starts to examine the remaining breast, draw cryptic ink lines around the surgical site, and discuss the operation. Do what you can to give them a private corner of the preop holding area for this purpose.

For the most part, this operation will be pretty tedious for you. Don't wake up the patient too early, because the actual suturing is followed by up to 20 minutes of ritualistic breast dressing during which the patient needs to remain asleep.

Liposuction

Description: The surgeon makes a small incision in the midst of the area to be suctioned and inserts an instrument that looks like the edge cleaner on your old Hoover vacuum. This instrument is rammed back and forth under the skin while connected to high-powered suction. Subcutaneous fat is loosened by the mechanical action and then removed by the vacuum.

Position:	Any
Estimated time:	60 minutes
Estimated blood loss:	300 ml; type and cross-match 2 units
Need for muscle relaxation:	None
Indicated monitors:	Standard
Postoperative analgesia:	II
Acceptable techniques:	GA, epidural, spinal

Comments: The patients are typically young and healthy and have lost some weight recently. Liposuction is done for aesthetic reasons to help even up the weight loss. Common areas for suctioning are the thighs, buttocks, abdomen, and flanks.

The surgeon will need to stand up the patient and mark out the areas to be trimmed before the operation begins. For modesty's sake, try to find them an out-of-the-way corner of the preop holding area for doing so, and hold off on the preop sedation.

Stimulation (and blood loss) are fairly intense but fairly brief.

You may have to turn the patient from front to back or side to side during the procedure—one reason that a regional technique may be easier and safer.

When the suction stops, the surgeon will need only a couple of minutes to close the small skin incision. Be prepared for a rapid finish.

Abdominoplasty ("Tummy Tuck")

Description: The surgeon excises a big piece of redundant skin and subcutaneous tissue from the patient's belly, then pulls the remaining edges together and closes.

Position:	Supine
Estimated time:	90 minutes
Estimated blood loss:	200 ml; type and screen
Need for muscle relaxation:	None
Indicated monitors:	Standard
Postoperative analgesia:	II
Acceptable techniques:	GA, spinal, epidural

Comments: The patient is generally young and otherwise healthy. Typically they will have lost a lot of weight recently, leaving a large redundant pannus. Every so often, though, in a scene from your worst nightmares, this operation is done for medical (as opposed to aesthetic) reasons on an enormously obese person who has a chronic skin infection, an impingement on breathing, or some other reason to need his or her gut removed.

The operation consists of a long skin incision, a delicate plastic surgery closure, and not much in between. The fatter the patient is to begin with, the longer the operation and the greater the blood loss.

Although regional anesthesia will be theoretically effective for this case, most of the time the patient just wants to go to sleep. General anesthesia for a large patient with a large pannus can be a challenge, to say the least. See the section on obesity in Chapter 1 for details.

Don't wake the patient up too quickly; the closure usually takes a long time.

Skin Graft

Description: The surgeon harvests a piece of skin from one portion of the body and staples or sutures it down over another. Full-thickness grafts are harvested with a scalpel and typically come from areas with redundant skin (like the groin). More common are split-thickness grafts, which are harvested from any flat area with a device that looks like a hand-held lawnmower.

Position:	Any
Estimated time:	60 minutes plus
Estimated blood loss:	200 ml plus; type and crossmatch 2 units
Need for muscle relaxation:	None
Indicated monitors:	Standard; consider Foley, A-line
Postoperative analgesia:	III
Acceptable techniques:	GETA, spinal, epidural

Comments: Skin grafts are most common in young, accident-prone individuals and are used to replace skin lost to burns and motor vehicle trauma. The patient will typically have been healthy to start with but may have traumatic injuries, infections, or multiple system failures by the time you get to meet him or her for this procedure.

Make sure you know where the graft is coming from as well as where it's going, especially if you are planning to use regional anesthesia. You may find yourself turning the patient from prone to supine, or vice versa, in the middle of the case.

Split-thickness graft harvest, which leaves behind enough skin to grow back on its own, is very stimulating for a short time. Securing the graft over the recipient site is not stimulating at all but may be time-consuming.

Blood loss can be brisk, both from the harvest site (despite the use of local epinephrine injections beforehand) and from "freshening" of the recipient site. The local epinephrine can add up to an impressive dose in a small child, causing arrhythmias, so make sure the surgeon knows what the acceptable limits are.

Fluid and heat loss can be considerable, especially in

the burned or pediatric patient.

Serious burns or trauma will lead to multiple grafting procedures as the patient is slowly pieced back together. Patients may be incredibly tolerant of narcotics by the fourth or fifth trip to the OR. Check their normal intake before starting the anesthetic, and plan to be generous.

Coexisting infections are common, and sterile technique is important.

The use of succinylcholine is contraindicated in many patients presenting for skin grafting, because of recent burns or trauma and concern with receptor up-regulation and the potential for a fatal hyperkalemic response.

Acute Burn Assessment

Description: The surgeon will bring the patient to the OR for a variety of purposes: correction of associated orthopedic injuries, débridement of severely burned tissue and clothing, fasciotomies to relieve compartment syndrome, and bronchoscopy to assess lung damage.

Position:	Any; may change during the procedure
Estimated time:	2 hours plus
Estimated blood loss:	300 ml plus; type and crossmatch 4 units
Need for muscle relaxation:	None
Indicated monitors:	Standard, Foley; consider A-line, central venous pressure
Postoperative analgesia:	IV
Acceptable techniques:	GETA

Comments: The patient will be in shock and will have an enormous volume requirement. There may be associated injuries including a cervical spine fracture, and a full stomach may complicate your induction.

Succinylcholine or high-dose vecuronium can be used for a rapid-sequence intubation. Succinylcholine does not pose a problem in the acutely burned patient.

The airway may be patent initially but may close rapidly due to swelling of burned mucosal tissue. Intubate early, and be prepared to use a smaller than normal endotracheal tube.

Hypoxia may be present due to carbon monoxide poisoning, lung damage and associated edema, and aspiration of soot particles. Bronchoscopy may be indicated to sort out these potential complications.

Tissue edema can lead to a compartment syndrome in any extremity, which must be relieved surgically. Circumferential burns of the thorax can cause a restrictive pulmonary deficit that will require an escharotomy to correct.

Severe postoperative pain, the need for multiple surgical procedures, and the potential for airway edema should all lead you to keep the patient intubated at the end of the procedure. Generally a high-dose narcotic technique will keep the patient happiest.

Strict sterile technique is indicated throughout, even though arterial and IV lines may have to be placed through severely burned tissue.

Volume, volume, volume!

Rotation Flap

Description: The surgeon frees up a hunk of muscle from the latissimus dorsi, quadriceps, trapezius, or pectoral muscle and swings it on a pedicle of nerve and blood vessels to fill some nearby defect created by trauma or cancer surgery.

Position:	Any
Estimated time:	3 hours
Estimated blood loss:	300 ml; type and cross-match 2 units
Need for muscle relaxation:	Required
Indicated monitors:	Standard, Foley; consider A-line
Postoperative analgesia:	III
Acceptable techniques:	GETA, epidural, combined

Comments: This operation can be done acutely as part of the cancer surgery that creates the hole or some time later when the traumatized tissue has declared its margins. Cancer patients are usually older and sicker, while trauma patients are younger and fundamentally more healthy, although associated injuries may make them sicker when you meet them.

A skin graft frequently accompanies this procedure to complete the coverage of the tissue defect.

Regional anesthesia, including combined technique, is highly encouraged. Sympatholysis and arterial dilatation will help the rotation flap to prosper. An epidural infusion will also provide great postoperative analgesia.

Keeping the patient warm is essential.

Do everything you can to maintain good tissue perfusion, including the earlier than normal use of blood products (after discussion with the surgeon, of course). If the urine output is falling, you should think about doing something sooner rather than later. The kidneys may be trying to tell you that the rotation flap is also underperfused. Listen to them!

Free Flap

Description: The surgeon removes a hunk of some muscle that the patient has more than enough of, such as the latissimus dorsi, taking care to identify its arterial and venous connections, and moves it to some other part of the body where it can fill a defect created by cancer surgery or trauma. The vessels are reconnected under a microscope, and the flap is covered over with a skin graft.

Position:	Any; may turn intraop
Estimated time:	6 hours
Estimated blood loss:	500 ml; type and cross-match 2 units
Need for muscle relaxation:	Required
Indicated monitors:	Standard, Foley, A-line; consider CVP line
Postoperative analgesia:	III
Acceptable techniques:	GETA, combined

Comments: The cancer patient may be older and sicker at baseline, but the trauma victim may have other associated injuries that complicate your anesthetic.

Microvascular anastomosis is a very finicky procedure that requires absolute stillness of the surgical field and a great deal of patience on your part.

The more perfusion the flap gets, the better. Use a regional anesthetic if possible, transfuse early, keep the patient warm, and keep the blood volume up. You should be shooting for a hematocrit of about 30.

Be wary of early flap failure necessitating a return to the OR for revision or reconstruction. Don't pull your epidural catheter until you're certain that the flap has "taken."

Pediatric Surgery

Robert M. Gantt

Pediatric cases come, like the patients, in all shapes and sizes. Virtually any operation that can be done in an adult can also be done in a child, but we don't intend to repeat this entire book in microcosm. Instead, we've selected the more common pediatric operations (some of which are also discussed in other chapters) and summarized them here.

Your patients may range in age from neonates all the way up to adolescents. Fortunately for you the effective dose of most anesthetic agents is the same—on a body weight basis—for all ages of patient. What *is* different about children is their reduced tolerance for apnea, a result of their increased metabolic rate and relatively smaller functional residual capacity (FRC). Young children have a fixed stroke volume (their heart works at capacity all the time) and tend to rely on their heart rate for cardiac output. Congenital cardiac anomalies may also complicate things immeasurably. Children also get cold very quickly, requiring you to keep the room temperature cranked up and to pay close attention to keeping them covered.

Inductions may be a challenge, especially in preschool children. Infants can be held down for monitor placement, IV starting, and induction, but as they get bigger this option becomes less attractive. The prototypical anesthetic induction in a 3-year-old involves cajoling the child away from the mother, carrying the child back into the OR, and "breathing him down" with nitrous oxide and halothane, all before applying any monitors (other than a precordial stethoscope) or establishing IV access. Those little amenities can be incorporated after a stable general anesthetic has been established. Rectal methohexital or oral midazolam can be given preoperatively to sedate the child and ease separation from the parents. IM injections (of ketamine, midazolam, or both) are reserved for the truly wild. School-age kids are usually a little more mature and may be able to cooperate with a mask induction or preoperative IV placement, if the provider is skilled. The recent introduction of EMLA cream to provide topical anesthesia for IV starts has made this process even easier. As the child gets older, separation becomes less of a concern, and you can proceed with inductions more reminiscent of your adult practice. Adolescents can be treated almost exactly like adults with some extra emphasis on anxiolysis. It is not unusual for the teenage patient, despite being NPO and appearing outwardly calm, to have a stomach full of churning acid.

Many pediatric operations are planned on a day-surgery basis. Going home within a few hours of the OR is a common practice, and your analgesic plan needs to take this into account. Little kids will not be able to describe their pain very well, and kids of all ages will become sedated very easily from narcotic preparations. We prefer to combine general anesthesia with local and regional anesthesia whenever possible, so that the patient never has the opportunity to become uncomfortable. This may take the form of a caudal or epidural block or simply having the surgeon infiltrate the wound with local as it is closed. For appropriate cases a caudal or other epidural catheter can be placed after the child is asleep, if your pediatric postop unit can manage it.

CT Scan

Description: The patient is placed on the gantry of the machine, taped in position, and then moved into the doughnut for the actual scan.

Position:	Usually supine
Estimated time:	45 minutes
Estimated blood loss:	Zero
Need for muscle relaxation:	None
Indicated monitors:	Standard
Postoperative analgesia:	I
Acceptable techniques:	GETA or heavy sedation

Comments: These patients may be children of any age with a wide range of congenital anomalies. (Or else why are you scanning them?) They may also be belligerent drunk motor vehicle accident victims from the ER or ICU. Your mission is to make the patient hold still for the scan in whatever way you can. A CT is less sensitive than an MRI but still requires stillness for each image.

Be wary of the patient who is "too sick to sedate": one with an intracranial mass and elevated intracranial pressure (ICP) who may become sedated all too easily. Sedation leads to respiratory depression, which leads to increased CO_2, which leads to an increase in ICP, which leads to more sedation, which leads to....here in the northern hemisphere these patients will have a tendency to go down the drain clockwise.

CTs can often be accomplished with heavy sedation but will sometimes require a general anesthetic. Access to the patient will be difficult because the scanner is in the way, so you'll want to make sure you're happy with the anesthetic before allowing the scan to start (and removing yourself from the radiation-filled immediate vicinity). A continuous infusion of propofol or methohexital is better than repeated IV doses.

If you are scanning an intubated patient from the ICU or ER, make sure you contact respiratory therapy beforehand to arrange for a ventilator in the CT scan room. You will probably not want to bring your anesthesia machine there for a patient who can be easily managed with IV agents. Also be careful with patient transport; use a

monitor and supplemental oxygen if the patient is still sedated postprocedure.

Some scans require the injection of iodinated contrast material, which has a propensity for causing allergic reactions. Have some epinephrine handy.

MRI Scan

Description: The child is anesthetized, shifted to the gantry of the MRI scanner, secured in place with all appropriate monitoring, and the scan is begun. Your credit cards are simultaneously erased. That is all.

Position:	Supine, with airway 10 feet from anesthesia provider
Estimated time:	60 minutes
Estimated blood loss:	Zero
Need for muscle relaxation:	None
Indicated monitors:	Standard
Postoperative analgesia:	I
Acceptable techniques:	GETA

Comments: Your patients will range all the way from otherwise normal but claustrophobic adults all the way down to severely anomalous infants.

Your mission is to make the patient hold still, since even the slightest movement might wash out the whole study. An MRI will almost always require a general anesthetic, partly because of the length and noise of the procedure, partly because the patient will be 6 feet up the tube of the machine from you. Make sure that all of your anesthetic equipment and monitors are MRI-compatible. Check oxygen and nitrous hookups and the availability of suction equipment. Do all of this *before* the patient arrives.

Typically you will induce general anesthesia, start your IV, and intubate the patient on the stretcher, then move the patient to the gantry of the scanner. Make sure you have enough slack in your tubes and wires to reach all the way into the machine. Spontaneous ventilation is something to strive for, as it gives you one more monitor of anesthetic depth and allows patients to titrate their own anesthetic depth when you are using a volatile anesthetic. Your end-tidal CO_2 monitor will be sipping through a 20-foot hose, so it won't be quantitatively accurate. However, a wave form does indicate continued ventilation.

Anything metallic is a big problem for the MRI scanner. Loose metal, like laryngoscope blades, scissors, or stethoscopes, will fly toward the magnet, damaging it or anything that gets in the way. Metal attached to the patient—ECG leads, hip pins, surgical staples—may heat up and cause an injury.

Not only will your credit cards erase (and your pocket calculator, and your watch, and your beeper), but your monitors may also have trouble with the magnetic fields. Oximeters must be specially constructed to work with the MRI, and capnometer and blood pressure cables will have to extend out of the room to their base units (make sure you can see the numbers from wherever you end up standing). An ECG may be completely impossible, and you may just have to do without.

There's nothing harmful about staying in the scan room with the patient (as far as we know now), although it can be pretty loud. You're closer if anything happens, and you can keep a better eye on the patient's ventilation. Just make sure you can see all the monitors you have, and ask the technician to let you know when the end of the scan is approaching.

Gadolinium is given as an IV contrast agent for some studies. As far as we can tell, it has no effect on your anesthetic.

Know how to get at the patient's airway in a hurry. There's normally a manual override lever that lets you pull the patient out of the scanner, if you have to. Know where this is and how it works.

Transport from the MRI to the PACU can be an exciting adventure. Provide supplemental oxygen, use a transport monitor if the patient is not wide awake, and carry emergency drugs and airway equipment with you.

Bilateral Myringotomy and Tubes (Ear Tubes) (BMTT)

Description: This staple of the ENT service is done through an operating microscope. A small incision is made in the eardrum and a little grommet is inserted to keep the hole open. Steroid ear drops are drizzled in to reduce swelling, the external ear is packed with cotton, and you're finished.

Position:	Supine
Estimated time:	15 minutes
Estimated blood loss:	Minimal
Need for muscle relaxation:	None
Indicated monitors:	Standard
Postoperative analgesia:	II; PO medications
Acceptable techniques:	GA

Comments: Typically done under mask anesthesia, with the patient breathing spontaneously, with the surgeon and anesthetist working together to stay out of each other's way.

In the routine pediatric case, you can skip the IV. Have IV starting material and an IM dose of succinylcholine and atropine handy, though, just in case you run into trouble.

Because this operation is done in children with chronic ear infections, you may have to accept a certain amount of sniffling and upper respiratory infection (URI) symptoms in your patient. Things that might make you cancel an elective hernia repair can be tolerated here, because the patient may never get any better. Usually you are able to maintain spontaneous ventilation and avoid an endotracheal tube. Still, be prepared for laryngospasm or other airway problems.

Tonsillectomy/Adenoidectomy

Description: Operating through the mouth, the surgeon scrapes the tonsillar and/or adenoidal tissue off the side of the pharynx, does something about the bleeding, and leaves.

Position:	Supine, bed turned away from the anesthetist
Estimated time:	45 minutes
Estimated blood loss:	50 ml; type and screen
Need for muscle relaxation:	Not necessary
Indicated monitors:	Standard
Postoperative analgesia:	II; PO medications, local injection by surgeon
Acceptable techniques:	GETA, local

Comments: Although previously performed mostly for tonsillitis, obstructive apnea is presently the leading reason for tonsillectomy/adenoidectomy. As with ear tubes, you may have to accept a certain amount of preoperative illness on the part of the patient, since they may have continuous URI/tonsillitis until this operation is done.

The surgeon will typically use a special tonsillar gag to hold the mouth open so the operation can be done. This gag holds your (oral) endotracheal tube in the midline of the tongue. Your circuit will typically approach from the patient's chest. Using a tube (RAE or Flexibend) designed to make a sharp corner southward from the mouth will help you avoid embarrassing tube kink incidents. Pay special attention to the airway; there will be several episodes of disconnection and reconnection of your circuit while the surgeon is getting the gag positioned.

The use of narcotics intraop in the obstructive-apnea tonsillectomy patient is controversial. You may want to discuss this issue with your staff anesthesiologist before proceeding.

Blood in the airway is a wonderful stimulant for laryngospasm. Make sure the surgeon has suctioned the patient thoroughly before you attempt to extubate.

If the surgeon uses a throat pack to keep blood out of the stomach, make sure it gets removed at the end of the case.

The surgeon may be planning to send the patient home on the day of surgery, but this approach may not always be reasonable, especially in young children who presented with obstructive apnea. Think about this issue as you drop off the child in the PACU.

Blood loss postoperatively can vanish invisibly into the stomach, leaving the patient significantly hypovolemic (and with a full stomach) when you take him or her back to the OR to correct the bleeding. This oral boards favorite situation is best approached with an IV rapid-sequence induction, after initial hydration, using an agent like ketamine that won't embarrass you.

Placing the IV in a location where it will stay in and then securing it well will make you look good if you do have to return to the OR. Avoid the antecubital fossa, if possible, and use an armboard or splint if the IV is near the wrist joint.

In cooperative adults this procedure can be done under local anesthesia alone, but not on any of us.

Circumcision

Description: "Just a little bit off the top, please." The surgeon pulls up the foreskin, cuts it off short, and sutures the loose edges together.

Position:	Supine
Estimated time:	30 minutes
Estimated blood loss:	Minimal
Need for muscle relaxation:	None
Indicated monitors:	Standard
Postoperative analgesia:	II; penile block by surgeons, caudal, oral medications
Acceptable techniques:	GA; local for adults and newborns

Comments: This procedure can usually be done as a mask general anesthetic, especially if your surgeon is swift. If the airway gets ugly, you can always intubate the child in the middle of the procedure. The surgeon is usually far enough away that you won't interfere with things.

A penile block by the surgeon at the end of the case is usually all the postoperative analgesia you need, although you may also choose to do a caudal block. If the child seems cranky postop despite good pain relief, consider the psychosocial issues involved, and refer him to a good Freudian psychiatrist.

Hypospadias Repair

Description: Typically performed in children, this operation is done to correct abnormalities in the terminal urethra and involves creating a conduit for urine that reaches all the way from the bladder to the distal meatus.

Position:	Supine
Estimated time:	2–3 hours
Estimated blood loss:	Minimal
Need for muscle relaxation:	None
Indicated monitors:	Standard
Postoperative analgesia:	II; PO medications, caudal or penile block
Acceptable techniques:	General, combined caudal/general

Comments: All of the usual pediatric concerns apply. The patient can be anywhere from a few months to a few years old.

There are usually no associated abnormalities accompanying hypospadias.

The length of surgery is related to the severity of the defect.

No Foley is available for monitoring urine output.

Older kids will have psychosocial issues associated with pain or surgical dressings involving their penises. This may cause increased regressive behavior, separation anxiety, and the like. A caudal block may prevent them from wanting to touch their penis, thereby avoiding interference with the dressings or contamination of the wound.

Reimplantation of Ureters

Description: This operation is performed, usually in pediatric patients, to correct a refluxing ureteral pelvic junction. The abdomen is opened through a midline incision, and the peritoneum and its contents are retracted superiorly. The ureters are identified and dissected free, cut at the bladder end, and then reattached in a reflux-proof fashion. Stents may be placed intraoperatively and are often left in place postoperatively.

Position:	Supine
Estimated time:	2–4 hours
Estimated blood loss:	50–100 ml; type and screen
Need for muscle relaxation:	Yes, for abdominal exposure
Indicated monitors:	Standard, Foley
Postoperative analgesia:	III; caudal or epidural, PCA if the patient is old enough
Acceptable techniques:	GETA, combined caudal/general

Comments: The usual pediatric considerations apply; patients can be of any age but are most commonly 2 to 5 years old. Ureteral reflux is not associated with any specific congenital syndromes, but a careful look for associated anomalies is important.

The operation often starts with a cystoscopy to confirm the existence of reflux and the need for the rest of the operation. Since the procedure can end abruptly at this point be careful not to overload the patient with anesthetics.

Urine output will be interrupted during the case but is a source of great concern to the urologists once their anastomoses are complete.

Pay attention to keeping the patients warm, especially if they're very young!

Umbilical Hernia Repair

Description: The skin is opened over the defect, the hernia sac is ligated, and the fascia is closed securely.

Position:	Supine
Estimated time:	60 minutes
Estimated blood loss:	30 ml
Need for muscle relaxation:	Required (may be optional for a small hernia)
Indicated monitors:	Standard
Postoperative analgesia:	II; local infiltration, caudal, PO medications
Acceptable techniques:	GA

Comments: These are usually healthy children, without associated problems, with funny bumps on their belly. They will typically be a couple of years old and will be having their surgery on a purely elective basis.

A mask induction is usually OK, with the IV placed after the child has quit squirming.

Umbilical hernias may appear deceivingly small, creating the temptation to complete the case under a mask anesthetic, particularly if the airway is easy. But when the surgeon stuffs a finger or two through that tiny defect and into the peritoneum and the patient subsequently bucks and squirts out a foot of intestine through the hole, you'll wish you had taken the anesthetic a little deeper and intubated the patient.

A caudal block with 0.50–0.75 ml/kg of 0.25% bupivacaine will provide excellent postoperative analgesia.

Try to keep the patient from bucking or straining with emergence as this will prematurely stress the surgical repair.

Pediatric Inguinal Hernia Repair

Description: The groin is opened, the hernia sac is identified and ligated, and the fascial layers are tightened up.

Position:	Supine
Estimated time:	60 minutes
Estimated blood loss:	Minimal
Need for muscle relaxation:	Not needed
Indicated monitors:	Standard
Postoperative analgesia:	II; caudal, local by surgeon, PO medications
Acceptable techniques:	GA, combined with caudal block, spinal in newborns

Comments: Hernias in children are frequently bilateral, so this procedure is often a bilateral repair.

The key is to avoid a lot of straining, coughing, and bucking with extubation. Unnecessarily stressing the surgical repair will get you rapidly into the doghouse.

A caudal block (done just after intubation) provides excellent postoperative pain relief and allows you to run a lighter anesthetic intraop. The standard mix is 0.50–0.75 ml/kg of 0.125–0.250% bupivacaine, typically without epinephrine.

Traction on the spermatic cord can cause some interesting arrhythmias, so pay attention to your ECG monitor. Bradycardia is most common and is best treated with IV atropine.

Mask inductions are fine, and mask anesthesia can be continued throughout the case if the surgery is going to be fast.

Pyloromyotomy

Description: Via a small upper abdominal incision the surgeon exposes the pylorus and then opens the muscular outer layer lengthwise. This incision is then closed crosswise, effectively relieving the pyloric stenosis, and everyone goes home.

Position:	Supine
Estimated time:	60 minutes
Estimated blood loss:	30 ml; type and screen
Need for muscle relaxation:	Required
Indicated monitors:	Standard
Postoperative analgesia:	III; IV medications, local infiltration by surgeon
Acceptable techniques:	GETA

Comments: These children (usually about 6 weeks old) will have been barfing for days at home. They will be dehydrated and will be at high risk for aspiration. You must insist that the child gets an IV placed in advance and is adequately hydrated (as judged by corrected electrolytes) before your rapid-sequence induction. Pyloromyotomy is a medical, not a surgical, emergency.

The radiologists will have thoughtfully filled the child's stomach with barium before sending him to the OR. Suction out the stomach via a nasogastric or orogastric tube before inducing anesthesia, and plan on a rapid-sequence induction in any case.

The patient may need a small amount of narcotics or some local anesthetic in the wound for postoperative analgesia.

Other than the pyloric stenosis, these patients are usually a normal size for their age and otherwise healthy.

Congenital Diaphragmatic Hernia

Description: The abdomen is opened, the abdominal contents are pulled back to their side of the diaphragm, the lung is carefully expanded with low pressures, and the patient is closed. Often a Silastic patch is needed to close the abdomen, which has not developed normally.

Position:	Supine
Estimated time:	3 hours
Estimated blood loss:	100 ml; type and cross-match 2 units
Need for muscle relaxation:	Required
Indicated monitors:	Standard
Postoperative analgesia:	IV; intravenous agents
Acceptable techniques:	GETA

Comments: This operation is performed at birth or very shortly thereafter in a typically very small, very sick patient. The neonate will typically be hypoxic, may have a patent ductus arteriosus or persistent fetal circulation as a result, and may have even been on extracorporeal membrane oxygenation (ECMO).

Intubation usually happens at birth, but check the tube position anyway. A nasogastric tube will be helpful in decompressing the stomach. It is very important to keep a close eye on airway pressures throughout the case. The underdeveloped lung on the side of the hernia is obviously at risk for rupture at too high an inflation pressure, and so is the relatively good lung on the other side. Pneumothorax in the closed side of the chest will lead rapidly to hemodynamic collapse.

Warmth is an enormous issue in these children, and careful fluid management, including transfusion, is important. Pay attention to what the surgeon is doing, and try to gauge how long the case is likely to continue.

Blood pressure fluctuations can occur with pressure on the mediastinum and vena cava. Keep an eye on the surgeons and let them know if they are leaning on something important.

The affected lung may not expand normally even when it has the pleura all to itself. Be gentle.

Postoperatively the patient will remain intubated, will have a chest tube in place, and will require many days of intensive care.

Thyroglossal Duct Cyst Excision

Description: A small incision is made in the neck and the cyst is removed. If the cyst has a patent connection to the oral cavity (which is not uncommon), the surgeon may also try to look in there to find and close the connection. For sure he will stick his finger in there from time to time to palpate the cyst and facilitate the excision.

Position:	Supine, head back, neck extended, arms tucked
Estimated time:	60 minutes
Estimated blood loss:	Minimal
Need for muscle relaxation:	None
Indicated monitors:	Standard
Postoperative analgesia:	II; local infiltration, PO medications
Acceptable techniques:	GETA

Comments: These patients are usually healthy children, without other congenital anomalies.

Mask inductions are OK for this procedure, with an IV placed after the child is asleep.

Local infiltration by the surgeon will provide excellent postoperative analgesia.

You and the surgeon may wind up competing for space in the child's mouth. Pay close attention to your endotracheal tube while the intraoral portion of the operation is underway. Consider a nasal endotracheal tube (ETT) if a significant amount of intraoral manipulation is likely.

Usually the postoperative airway is no great concern, but if there is an unusual amount of swelling or bleeding in the neck a problem could develop. Take this into account before extubating the patient.

Orthopedic Surgery for Cerebral Palsy

Description: This procedure is different for each patient, depending on the specific needs of the child and the long-term surgical plan. Bilateral osteotomies (to straighten the bones) and tendon releases (to allow full range of motion of the joints) are common components.

Position:	Supine, rarely lateral
Estimated time:	3 hours
Estimated blood loss:	200 ml; type and cross-match 2 units
Need for muscle relaxation:	Required
Indicated monitors:	Standard, Foley
Postoperative analgesia:	III; caudal or epidural block, intravenous agents
Acceptable techniques:	GETA

Comments: These patients are often quite severely deformed, which may present you with a variety of anesthetic problems. Line placements may be difficult, and patience and attention to detail will be required when positioning the patient on the operating table.

Your technique for induction will be based on the individual patient. Some children will be calm enough to allow a mask induction prior to IV placement; others will require an IV placement first. Some children may be so severely uncooperative (perhaps due to months and years of ongoing medical care) that an IM injection of ketamine or midazolam is needed.

Blood loss can be substantial in the larger procedures of this type. Talk with the surgeon beforehand and try to get a handle on what is intended. If bleeding is likely to be an issue, you may want to place an arterial line after induction. Pay close attention to the patient's temperature, and keep the room as warm as necessary.

Frequent fluoroscopy is common. Wear your lead.

When the procedure is over it's not really done. Most of these operations end with placement of a bilateral hip spica cast, which can take up to an hour and involves a lot of patient manipulation. Don't let your anesthesia wear off too soon.

Patent Ductus Arteriosus (PDA) Ligation

Description: The surgeon makes a small left lateral thoracotomy, retracts or packs the left lung out of the way, and identifies the patent ductus. This is then ligated twice, and the chest and skin are closed.

Position:	Right lateral decubitus
Estimated time:	45 minutes
Estimated blood loss:	20 ml plus; type and crossmatch 2 units
Need for muscle relaxation:	Required
Indicated monitors:	Standard
Postoperative analgesia:	IV, local infiltration, IV medications
Acceptable techniques:	GETA

Comments: This operation may be done on neonates (especially premature) in the OR or neonatal ICU, or on larger kids of any age. The PDA is apt to be symptomatic in the former group, with congestive heart failure exacerbating underlying pulmonary disease. In the latter group, it is apt to be an incidental finding in an otherwise healthy patient. The untreated PDA will often not become symptomatic until adulthood, when the left-to-right shunt results in cardiac failure or even pulmonary hypertension. Any patient with a PDA is at increased risk for endocarditis and paradoxical embolization (some of the reasons to do this surgery).

Lung isolation and selective ventilation are not required for what is often a brief case, which is good because the technology for one-lung ventilation in children is nonexistent. About all you can do, if it becomes an issue, is push your endotracheal tube down into the right mainstem bronchus. This will take out the right upper lobe, of course, but most children will tolerate this for a short time as long as there are no other significant cardiopulmonary defects. However, do not try this with neonates; they don't tolerate it.

Neonates requiring PDA ligation will probably have already been intubated. Some of these patients can be quite premature and weigh less than 1 kg! An increase in the FIO_2 may be necessary intraoperatively. However, retrolental fibroplasia is associated with hyperoxia, so titrate the FIO_2 to the desired SaO_2. Other concerns with these patients are transport, maintenance of body temperature, positioning (e.g., ETT stability, prevention of bone and skin trauma), and avoidance of overdosage of fluids and drugs. Intraoperatively, the aorta or left pulmonary artery may be ligated (rather than the PDA). The disappearance of a pulse oximeter trace from the lower extremity can tip you off to the former. Neonates will almost uniformly continue to require ventilatory support in the immediate postop period.

Older children coming for PDA ligation can be managed according to your usual pediatric policy, with a mask induction and subsequent IV placement. Blood loss should be minimal, although the potential for disaster is obviously great.

The surgeon will seal the chest over a small suction catheter, then aspirate and remove it before closing the skin. With luck and careful intraop handling of the lung, there will be no air leak and no significant pneumothorax. A chest tube is often placed in adults or when significant lung damage has occurred.

Postoperatively, the patient will usually be watched in an ICU, both for pneumothorax monitoring and pain control. Local infiltration of the wound by the surgeon will help with the latter issue; 8 hours of postoperative comfort will usually get you to the point where the child can take oral medications. Bigger kids can get epidural catheters and stay on a continuous infusion until their pain has diminished, or get a single dose of caudal morphine.

Vascular Surgery

Vascular surgery patients are generally very sick. Unlike cardiac anesthesia where the patient with the bad heart stands a chance of being better at the end of the operation, the patient with the aortic aneurysm and the bad heart will still have the bad heart.

Hemodynamically, you will frequently be confronted with the choice of benefiting the heart (by reducing the heart rate) or benefiting the body (by working the heart with inotropes). Your preoperative assessment should focus on both the patient's cardiac risk and the risk of hypoperfusion to other tissues, including the brain, gut, kidneys, and lower extremities. Check the blood pressure in both arms before starting; not infrequently, there will be a significant difference from one side to the other.

Regional and combined anesthesia are common in vascular cases. The sympathectomy induced by an epidural or spinal anesthetic will be beneficial to the perfusion of the lower extremities but may make blood pressure support necessary. Using an epidural or spinal catheter to maintain anesthesia confers another advantage as well: In the relatively common circumstance of a return to the OR in the immediate postoperative period, the prior placement of a catheter can avoid the thorny decision of whether the benefit of doing a regional anesthetic is outweighed by the risk of the procedure in an anticoagulated patient.

Vascular anesthesia will give you the opportunity to learn about some new drugs. Heparin is given whenever an artery is clamped to prevent clot formation around the clamp and in the downstream vessel. The usual dose is 5,000 units IV, and you should record the time when you give it. Notify the surgeon after 1 hour so that more heparin can be given if the procedure is going to continue for much longer. When the arterial work is done the heparin can either be allowed to resolve spontaneously or protamine can be given to reverse it. One milligram of protamine reverses 100 units of active heparin (based on the time since the last dose). In some cases, of course, the surgeon will want the patient to remain anticoagulated. An infusion of heparin or low molecular weight dextran can be used. Dextran is a substance that binds to red cell surfaces, making them more slippery and less likely to clot on fresh suture lines. Dextran is highly immunogenic, however, and your infusion should always be preceded by a dose of dextran-1 (Promit), an even lower molecular weight dextran that binds to antibodies without triggering a reaction.

What you get out of vascular surgery: arterial lines, pulmonary artery catheters, thoracic epidurals (if you're aggressive), combined technique, and a comfort level for really sick patients. What your staff gets out of it: chest pain and indigestion.

Arteriovenous (AV) Fistula Creation

Description: The surgeon makes a couple of incisions in the forearm, exposing a likely-looking vein and artery, and then joins them with a special graft.

Position:	Supine, arm out
Estimated time:	90 minutes
Estimated blood loss:	100 ml; type and screen
Need for muscle relaxation:	Not needed
Indicated monitors:	Standard
Postoperative analgesia:	II
Acceptable techniques:	GETA, arm block, local plus sedation

Comments: The patients will usually be sick from a renal standpoint but not so sick that they give you much trouble. You should check their labs carefully, especially their creatinine and potassium levels, to find out how urgently they need to be dialyzed. Most patients for this procedure will be stable, since the unstable ones get a big catheter in the subclavian and a few weeks of buffing before coming for their AV fistula.

We've had good luck doing axillary blocks for these cases, since any nerves you miss can be easily topped up by the surgeon on the field. The surgeon will also appreciate the effect of sympatholysis on the artery being sewn. The transarterial approach is not recommended, just in case you get really unlucky and screw up the vessel.

If you do find yourself doing a general anesthetic, remember to use drugs that are not metabolized by the kidneys. Pancuronium, for example, is probably a bad idea.

Heparin is given before clamping the artery. Significant bleeding is usually uncommon since the vessels are superficial and easily controlled. Protamine is therefore seldom necessary.

You may also get to do this case as a repeat, since fistula failure is not uncommon. Unlike most "redo" surgeries, the AV fistula reconstruction is no worse than the original.

Vein Stripping/Saphenous Vein Ligation

Description: Through numerous small stab incisions in the skin the patient's varicose veins are excised. In addition, the saphenous vein is often ligated at its junction with the femoral.

Position:	Supine, prone, or both; Trendelenburg to shrink veins
Estimated time:	60 minutes
Estimated blood loss:	100 ml; type and screen
Need for muscle relaxation:	Not needed
Indicated monitors:	Standard
Postoperative analgesia:	II
Acceptable techniques:	GA, epidural, spinal, local

Comments: These patients are usually young and healthy. Although there are medical indications for this procedure (pain, central embolization), the overwhelming majority of these cases are done for cosmesis.

Depending on the location of the operative veins, the patient may have to be turned intraoperatively from supine to prone. Make sure you don't lose anything important in the process (like the airway, for instance).

Typically the surgeon will want to mark out the offending veins before the patient goes to sleep. Since that is best done with the patient standing, make sure the surgeon has had a chance to do so before sedating, anesthetizing, or tangling up the patient with an IV.

Limited procedures can be done under local anesthesia, but any patient receiving more than a few incisions should get a serious anesthetic.

Carotid Endarterectomy

Description: The side of the neck is opened and the carotid bifurcation is dissected free. Clamps are placed above and below, and the artery is opened lengthwise. The atherosclerotic plaque is scraped off the vessel wall and the artery is closed, sometimes incorporating a small patch of Goretex or harvested vein. Closure of the neck is rapid.

Position:	Semi-Fowler's, head turned, neck extended, arms tucked
Estimated time:	150 minutes
Estimated blood loss:	200 ml; type and cross-match 2 units
Need for muscle relaxation:	Helpful for the anesthetic
Indicated monitors:	Standard, A-line; consider Foley
Postoperative analgesia:	II
Acceptable techniques:	GETA or regional (deep and superficial cervical plexus block)

Comments: The leading cause of death after carotid endarterectomy is myocardial infarction. Your patient will have coronary disease in addition to carotid disease; make sure you know how much and how much it limits him. Stroke following arterial occlusion is another major concern. It can happen from inadequate collateral flow through the circle of Willis or as the result of embolization of debris from the artery when it is clamped.

Brain function can be monitored intraop by having the patient awake or by the use of raw EEG or compressed or digital brain wave monitoring. Changes in the EEG or loss of function in the awake patient is treated by raising the blood pressure to improve collateral flow. In anesthetized patients the surgeon may place a Silastic shunt to carry blood around the portion of artery being operated on. Some surgeons will shunt every patient, just in case.

Vagal reactions to carotid bulb manipulation are best handled by injection of local anesthesia on the field. Make sure the surgeon has it ready.

The case can be done as a GETA, which imposes the extra risk of induction and intubation on the patient and makes it harder to assess neurologic status intraop but guarantees the surgeon a quiet field and leaves you well prepared to deal with emergencies. It can also be done under regional anesthesia with the patient awake. This provides early warning of neurologic complications but may cause trouble if the patient does not tolerate the surgery or if some crisis develops (such as uncontrolled bleeding). Your access to the patient's airway is minimal once the surgery starts. Most surgeons (and institutions) will be preferentially comfortable with one technique or the other. You are best advised to do what the surgeon desires, since this is a high-stakes operation where good karma is important.

In either case, a carotid endarterectomy is almost painless postoperatively. Since the surgeon will be looking for a quick wake-up, make sure you don't overdose the patient. The surgeon will also tell you where the blood pressure should be during and after the case. Within reason, we generally go along.

An infusion of low molecular weight dextran is commonly requested perioperatively to decrease the chance of thrombus forming on the fresh vascular suture lines. When starting the dextran, remember to give an ampule (50 ml) of dextran-1 first to prevent an anaphylactic response.

Bleeding in the neck is not unusual postoperatively, because of the use of heparin and dextran. You should treat this as a serious problem, since airway edema can develop very quickly with a hematoma. Intubate early, use a smaller than normal tube, and be prepared to open the neck and decompress the hematoma as soon as possible.

Aortobifemoral Bypass Graft (AFB or ABF)

Description: This procedure is done to relieve claudication and impaired circulation to the pelvis and lower extremities. The belly and both groins are opened, the gut is mobilized out of the way, the aorta is exposed and cross-clamped, and a bifurcated graft is sewn to the aorta (either end to end or end to side) and into both common femoral arteries (after tunneling). The clamps are removed, the legs are reperfused, and all the wounds are closed.

Position:	Supine
Estimated time:	5 hours
Estimated blood loss:	1,000 ml plus; type and crossmatch 4 units; use cell saver
Need for muscle relaxation:	Required
Indicated monitors:	Standard, Foley, A-line, CVP/PA line
Postoperative analgesia:	III
Acceptable techniques:	GETA, combined

Comments: These patients tend to have disseminated atherosclerosis, including their coronary and carotid arteries. Fortunately for you, they will also have well-developed collateral vessels to their pelvis so that the effects of clamping and unclamping the aorta are mitigated. This operation will take longer than a straight tube graft for an aortic aneurysm but is similar in many details. You should read the next section on abdominal aortic aneurysm resection in addition to this one.

Unlike in a straight tube graft, in this case the surgeon will reperfuse the legs individually as he or she finishes each distal graft. Which leg causes the greater hemodynamic perturbation with opening will vary from patient to patient. The larger surface area is reperfused with the first leg, since left-to-right collaterals effectively perfuse the entire pelvis from either iliac vessel. The second leg, on the other hand, will have been cold longer and will have built up more of a toxic load than the first.

Either one will be less severe than opening an aortic tube graft, however.

Perfusion of the distal extremities is the goal of this operation—and the biggest concern. Using an epidural anesthetic will probably improve flow, but using a lot of phenylephrine will probably worsen it. If blood pressure support is required, consider the use of dopamine or a similar inotropic agent.

Central access is clearly required because of the high likelihood that you will be infusing vasoactive substances at some point. Whether you use a central venous pressure or a pulmonary artery monitor is a matter of institutional preference, patient illness, and personal experience.

Abdominal Aortic Aneurysm (AAA) Resection—Infrarenal

Description: The belly is opened, the guts are mobilized to the side, and the aorta is dissected free. Clamps are placed above and below the aneurysm, which is then opened lengthwise. A tube of Dacron or Goretex is then used to bypass the aneurysmal section. The clamps are removed, reperfusing the lower body, and the aneurysm, peritoneum, and fascia are closed over the graft.

Position:	Supine; rarely right lateral decubitus
Estimated time:	4 hours
Estimated blood loss:	1,000 ml; type and crossmatch 4 units; use cell saver
Need for muscle relaxation:	Required
Indicated monitors:	Standard, Foley, A-line, CVP/PA line
Postoperative analgesia:	III
Acceptable techniques:	GETA, combined

Comments: Knowing the likely hemodynamic course of the operation will help you anticipate the path and keep you from overreacting to perturbations. The blood pressure will usually go down with induction, up with intubation, down with manipulation of the gut, up sharply with cross-clamping, but then right down with bleeding, and then down even more sharply when the cross-clamp comes off.

The most impressive bleeding comes when the aneurysm is opened and is caused by back-bleeding lumbar vessels in the rear wall of the aneurysm. These vessels can only be oversewn from the inside and may bleed freely until then.

Mannitol (12.5 g) is given routinely just before clamping and just before unclamping. Even with the proximal clamp applied below the level of the renal arteries, there is a substantial decrease in renal blood flow as well as the potential for knocking emboli into the kidneys. Urine output should be followed closely, and furosemide and low-dose dopamine should be added to the mannitol if necessary.

Using an epidural catheter as part of the anesthetic can smooth out a lot of the bumps in the course of the case, although the presence of a sympathectomy can make it difficult to determine the patient's true volume status.

If the operation goes well the patient may be a candidate for extubation in the OR. If any complications arise, if the case runs long and you end up giving a large volume load, or if you think pain relief may not be adequate, then it is probably more prudent to leave the patient intubated until things have stabilized postoperatively.

Abdominal Aortic Aneurysm (AAA) Resection—Suprarenal

Description: Same as the infrarenal aorta, except that the proximal clamp goes on higher up and some extra suturing is required to attach the celiac, superior mesenteric, and left and right renal arteries to the aortic graft.

Position:	Partial right lateral decubitus, thoracoabdominal approach
Estimated time:	6 hours
Estimated blood loss:	2,000 plus; type and crossmatch 8 units; fresh-frozen plasma, platelets, cell saver, big IV!
Need for muscle relaxation:	Required
Indicated monitors:	Standard, Foley, PA, A-line; consider transesophageal echocardiography
Postoperative analgesia:	IV
Acceptable techniques:	GETA

Comments: In the abdomen, this case is like an AAA, only more so. In the chest things get much more complicated. The abdominal version is here; the thoracic version is in the chapter on cardiac surgery. Some specific concerns:

1. Cardiac—The heart may take a big hit from the high cross-clamping. Have some nitroprusside running to help reduce the pressure before the clamp goes on. Be very prepared for clamp release.
2. Renal—The beans are taking a hit. Use mannitol before the clamp goes on and before it comes off. Plan to use a furosemide/mannitol or dopamine infusion postop. Some surgeons will ice the kidneys or fill them with a cold perfusing solution intraop.
3. Gut—Ischemia can only be minimized by fast surgery. Gut ischemia adds greatly to the dive the patient will take when the clamp comes off.

4. Clotting—Coagulopathies are common due to the large exposed surface of graft (which eats platelets) and the exclusion of the liver and spleen from the circulation when the clamp is on. Use colloid only for replacement, and go with fresh-frozen plasma and platelets early.

5. Spinal cord—Ischemia is common with a high aortic clamp. (Remember the artery of Adamkiewicz?) Function can be monitored with somatosensory evoked potentials, but this has been shown to be only marginally useful. A spinal drain may be helpful to drain cerebrospinal fluid during clamping and maintain a constant spinal pressure less than 20 mm Hg, thereby preserving an adequate spinal cord perfusion pressure. Some centers are now experimenting with cooling the spinal cord, as well.

6. There's just no substitute for fast surgery.

Thrombectomy/Embolectomy

Description: This procedure is typically done for a lower extremity vascular occlusion, either in a native vessel or a bypass graft. The vessel is accessed above the occlusion—typically in the groin—and a thin Fogarty catheter is passed down the vessel as far as possible. The balloon on the end is then inflated and the catheter reeled in. On a good day, all of the obstructing clot is pulled out with it. On a bad day, you'll need to look at the next section: distal revascularization.

Position:	Supine
Estimated time:	60 minutes
Estimated blood loss:	200 ml plus; type and crossmatch 2 units
Need for muscle relaxation:	Not required
Indicated monitors:	Standard; consider A-line
Postoperative analgesia:	II
Acceptable techniques:	GETA, spinal, epidural, or combined

Comments: These are the usual old, sick vascular patients, usually in acute pain from their ischemic extremity. The case may be an emergency if the occlusion is significant enough, meaning that the patient will have a full stomach and may not be medically buffed.

A simple thrombectomy is an easy procedure. Very often, though, it degenerates into a femoropopliteal or other bypass graft and becomes a long and tedious case. Bear this in mind as you are making your anesthetic plan. The few extra minutes an epidural takes over a spinal may pay off 2 hours later when the surgeon is still at it.

On the other hand, the patient may already be anticoagulated, and any regional procedure may be contraindicated. A simple thrombectomy can be done under local anesthesia but for anything more complicated than that, GETA should be considered.

If the patient has had a painful limb and has been unable to sleep, they may nod off very easily following a successful regional blockade. Bear this in mind before slugging them with the midazolam.

Regional anesthesia will improve blood flow to the affected vessels; phenylephrine may worsen it. The surgeon will typically ask for an infusion of either heparin or low molecular weight dextran at the end of the case. If you start the dextran infusion, remember to give the 50 ml of dextran-1 (Promit) first!

Distal Revascularization— Femoropopliteal, Femorotibial, Popliteotibial, etc.

Description: An occluded section of artery is bypassed using either a Goretex tube (if it crosses no joints) or a section of vein harvested from a leg or arm and stripped of its valves. Adequate distal perfusion is then assessed by color, temperature, angiography, pulse volume resistance (PVR), or Doppler flow.

Position:	Supine
Estimated time:	3 hours plus
Estimated blood loss:	500 ml plus; type and crossmatch 4 units
Need for muscle relaxation:	Not necessary
Indicated monitors:	Standard, Foley, A-line; consider pulmonary artery catheter
Postoperative analgesia:	III
Acceptable techniques:	GETA, epidural, spinal, or combined

Comments: The patient will be the typical high-risk vasculopath and should be assumed to have coronary artery disease until proven otherwise. Exercise tolerance will typically be zero, since the patient's claudication makes exercise impossible.

Regional anesthesia is good for blood flow and may be easier than general in many of these cases. Because the procedure will frequently go longer than planned (as the surgeon revises and revises and revises) you should use a single-shot spinal only if you trust the surgeon to keep the case short.

You may wish to pause and consider the patient's coagulation status before initiating a regional anesthetic. These patients are often heparinized preoperatively and may have elevated clotting and bleeding times. A case can be made that the risk of a general anesthetic outweighs the risk of an epidural hematoma in this population, but that is an issue you should discuss with your staff anesthesiologist beforehand.

Bleeding is never very dramatic but can accumulate to a fair amount over time.

The surgeon will typically request a heparin or low molecular weight dextran infusion postoperatively to encourage the graft to remain patent. If you start the dextran you must remember to give an ampule (50 ml) of dextran-1 first to prevent an anaphylactic response.

Femoral Exploration

Description: The surgeon opens the patient's groin over the site of the bleeding and carefully dissects down around the femoral artery. When adequate control has been obtained, the artery can be clamped and the specific problem addressed. Once a patent, nonleaking lumen has been reestablished, the clamp is removed, hemostasis is obtained, and the groin is closed.

Position:	Supine
Estimated time:	60 minutes
Estimated blood loss:	200 ml; type and cross-match 2 units
Need for muscle relaxation:	None
Indicated monitors:	Standard, 5-lead; consider A-line
Postoperative analgesia:	II
Acceptable techniques:	GETA, spinal, local

Comments: Ah, the groin shambles! So called because this case often comes to you on an emergency basis in a very sick patient with a veritable cloud of hand-wringing cardiologists and/or radiologists in attendance. The surgical problem is a pseudoaneurysm or uncontrollable bleeding from the femoral artery, typically caused by catheterization for great vessel or cardiac angiography. Since patients were presumably in need of the radiologic procedure that created the problem in the groin, they will probably not be in the best condition for you. At best they'll have vascular disease with the suspicion of coronary involvement. At worst they'll have just had a major cardiac procedure, such as a percutaneous transluminal coronary angioplasty, atherectomy, or laser atherolysis. If the procedure didn't work, the patient may be having impressive cardiac ischemia on arrival to the OR. This also applies to those patients in whom the femoral disruption was caused by placement or removal of an intra-aortic balloon pump.

Your job therefore consists of rapidly anesthetizing a hemodynamically unstable (or potentially so) cardiac patient who may be anemic, anticoagulated, and in pain. This sort of scariness is why some of these procedures get done as locals.

Once the patient is anesthetized the vascular surgeon's job is easy. Open the groin, correct the bleeding, and go home. Occasionally a patch of Goretex or harvested vein is necessary to close the artery without constricting it too much. This may make the case a little more tedious for you but will more likely just give you time to catch your breath.

Hemodynamic instability is common both from the patient's underlying coronary disease and from blood loss. An arterial line is recommended in this situation, to keep close track of the blood pressure while you are infusing nitroglycerin, heparin, phenylephrine, dopamine, or whatever.

Even though there will be a great commotion accompanying the patient to the OR, be obsessive about transferring from bed to bed. Losing IV lines will only make things worse!

Above Knee Amputation (AKA)

Description: A large scalpel is used to cut through the soft tissue above the knee, then a saw is used on the femur. Obvious vessels are ligated, everything else is electrocauterized, and the remaining muscle is folded up over the bone stump and loosely sutured.

Position:	Supine
Estimated time:	60 minutes
Estimated blood loss:	300 ml; type and cross-match for 2 units
Need for muscle relaxation:	Not needed
Indicated monitors:	Standard, 5-lead
Postoperative analgesia:	III
Acceptable techniques:	Spinal or epidural is highly recommended

Comments: These patients are usually older, sicker, and very unhappy about the need for an amputation. Except for the rare trauma patient, this operation is typically performed on diabetic vascular patients who may have failed distal bypass grafting. They will almost certainly be at risk for myocardial ischemia as well.

A great deal of bleeding can occur in a very short time but is usually rapidly controlled. During the Civil War there were legendary tales of the 11-second AKA, but most of your surgeons will take a little longer.

Regional anesthesia is highly recommended as a means of preventing phantom limb pain, which normally has an incidence of up to 70% in these patients. Published studies have looked at 24 hours of preoperative epidural blockade followed by 48 hours postop and have demonstrated a significantly lower incidence of subsequent phantom limb pain. Most facilities don't have the resources to go that far, but simply doing the case under a regional anesthetic seems to be almost as effective.

Be aware of the social issues involved. Provide generous sedation and don't make insensitive remarks!

Below Knee Amputation (BKA)

Description: Pretty much like you'd imagine. The soft tissue is cut and cauterized while any vessel large enough to have a name is ligated. The tibia and fibula are cut across with a saw and then the muscles are folded up into a flap and sutured.

Position:	Supine
Estimated time:	75 minutes
Estimated blood loss:	200 ml; type and cross-match 2 units
Need for muscle relaxation:	Not needed
Indicated monitors:	Standard, 5-lead
Postoperative analgesia:	III
Acceptable techniques:	Regional anesthesia highly recommended

Comments: BKA patients are typically elderly diabetics with failed femorotibial bypass grafts. They are at high risk for coronary artery disease and perioperative myocardial ischemia.

Surgically these cases are more challenging than AKAs and are usually done by a more senior resident.

Bleeding may be brisk for a few minutes but is usually easily controlled. A tourniquet may be placed, just in case, but is rarely used.

Regional anesthesia will reduce the incidence of phantom limb pain postoperatively and is usually preferred for this procedure. Epidural infusions postoperatively are also good.

Don't do a leg block if the patient has had vascular surgery on that limb. The surgeon will not thank you if you impale the femoral graft with your block needle.

Bear in mind that this operation will be psychologically very difficult for the patient. Titrate your sedation to the patient's condition, of course, but be prepared to be generous.

Toe or Foot Amputation

Description: The toe or foot is amputated using a sharp knife, an electrocautery, and a saw or bone cutter. Enough of a flap is created to cover the bone.

Position:	Supine
Estimated time:	90 minutes
Estimated blood loss:	100 ml; type and screen
Need for muscle relaxation:	None
Indicated monitors:	Standard, 5-lead
Postoperative analgesia:	II
Acceptable techniques:	Regional (spinal or leg/ankle block) recommended

Comments: The patient is the usual vasculopathic problem, often with a failed bypass graft in the same leg and usually afflicted with diabetes, coronary artery disease, and chronic obstructive pulmonary disease.

A foot amputation (transmetatarsal amputation) typically takes longer than either an above-knee or below-knee leg amputation, as the anatomy of the foot is quite complex. Toe amputations, on the other hand, can be much faster.

Regional anesthesia is recommended because it may help reduce the incidence of phantom limb pain postoperatively. Any leg or ankle block must avoid previous surgical sites.

Blood loss is usually minimal. A tourniquet may be placed, just in case, but will typically only be inflated in a real crisis. The surgeon will usually prefer to see what is bleeding and what is not so that all of the nonperfused tissue can be removed.

As with any amputation, psychological issues may be very important. Be sensitive to the patient's depression.

Neurosurgery

Paul A. Pudimat

Neuroanesthesia is a high-stakes game for those who like watching the surgeon mess around with that black box of physiology, the brain. You never know quite what you're going to get when you wake up craniotomy patients. Most of the time they're fine, but every so often you lose something—like all of 1974 (what the heck, it was a boring year anyway) or the ability to speak (oops!) or breathe (bigger oops). And it's not unusual to get your shot at neuroanesthesia at night, on an emergency basis, or in a situation where you can't be sure if the patient even remembered 1974 to begin with.

Waking up the patient promptly is an essential skill since the neurosurgeon is even more interested than you are in how the patient is going to emerge. Even in relatively simple spinal cases, a crisp awakening is highly desired so the surgeon can do the squeeze-my-hands-wiggle-your-toes routine.

Inductions are exciting, too. In craniotomies you must be concerned with keeping the intracranial pressure (ICP) low, the blood pressure under control, and the heart rate adequate. You must also stand by while the surgeons position the head in a three-point holder that looks like some distant descendant of Grandpa's ice tongs, using stainless steel "pins" that screw through the skin and into the cranium.

In spinal cases you are very often dealing with a bad airway and a complex intubation, followed by an exciting period of turning the patient over, losing all your monitors, positioning the patient, repositioning the patient, and worrying about the fate of your endotracheal tube.

Intraoperatively you can relax—until something happens, that is. Sudden bleeding in the brain can ruin your whole day, even if you have the recommended large-bore IV access. A venous air embolism can be even more exciting. Hypertension is common at the end of the procedure, especially as you shoot for that crisp wake-up, and may require specific pharmacology to correct.

Almost all neurosurgery cases are characterized by poor access to the endotracheal tube, either because the patient is in a funny position or because the head is in pins and draped off from you. Learn to take care when securing the tube to avoid embarrassment down the road.

What do you get out of it? Practice with the cervical spine patient, fiberoptic intubations, exposure to neurologic monitoring, arterial lines, and maybe a long-line CVP or two.

THE INTRACRANIAL PRESSURE GAME

ICP is one of those things that neuroanesthetists spend a lot of time thinking about, along with Caribbean island fantasies and winning a million in the lottery. The reason is that if the intracranial pressure gets too high, the brain tissue starts to get squeezed; squeeze the brain too hard and it can herniate, which is not good, or just stay where it is and asphyxiate, which is also not good. Most of the time in most people, excessive ICP is not a problem; ICP stays at a comfortable 10 mm Hg and doesn't change much. In people who need brain surgery, on the other hand, it's often a big deal.

The reason it's such a big deal is that the higher the ICP, the lower the cerebral perfusion pressure (CPP). Perfusion is as important to the brain as it is to any other tissue and is equally hard to measure. CPP is roughly equivalent to the mean arterial pressure less CVP or ICP, whichever is higher. Keeping the ICP under control is therefore critical to keeping the patient's neurons well perfused.

Brain tumors displace tissue, raising pressure. Extravascular blood, as from a hemorrhaging vessel, also displaces tissue and raises pressure. Not only is this bad for the brain, but the effect is worst right around the area of the pathology where the surgeon is going to have to retract the brain—putting more pressure on it—to fix the primary problem. A swollen brain will make it more difficult to get at the pathology—hence your desire to lower the ICP, particularly when the surgeons are actually approaching the area of interest.

Lowering the ICP can be accomplished in a number of ways. Hyperventilation (to a $PaCO_2$ of 25–30 mm Hg) will decrease ICP, as will the administration of diuretics like mannitol and furosemide. Steroids will shrink the area around a tumor but have little effect on collections of blood, as from a leaking aneurysm. Drainage of cerebrospinal fluid (CSF) via either a lumbar intrathecal catheter or a ventriculostomy will also shrink the brain. Apply these therapies when the surgeon asks you for them.

Lowering the cerebral metabolic rate ($CMRO_2$) by using thiopental or other barbiturates will indirectly decrease cerebral blood flow and reduce the size of the brain while simultaneously increasing its tolerance for hypoxia. Decreasing the patient's temperature will have the same effect.

Anesthetizing the patient with an elevated ICP is a challenge because the last thing you want to do is make it go any higher. Yet rises in ICP are associated with anxiety, with laryngoscopy and tracheal intubation, with putting in the pins for the head holder, and with the surgical incision. Oversedate the patient, on the other hand, and you may raise his or her CO_2, raising the ICP. The answer for this conundrum typically involves a deep narcotic level achieved with a bolus and then an infusion of a synthetic narcotic, a lot of thiopental (which is good for the brain because it lowers the metabolic rate and hence the oxygen consumption of brain tissue), and as little time as possible spent in a heavily sedated state. (In other words, you want to go from lightly sedated to intubated and hyperventilated without much in between.) Keep the anesthetic light throughout the case and be prepared to use a lot of antihypertensive medicine when you turn the anesthetic off at the end.

CT Scan

Description: The patient is placed on the gantry of the machine, taped in position, and then moved into the doughnut for the actual scan.

Position:	Usually supine
Estimated time:	45 minutes
Estimated blood loss:	Zero
Need for muscle relaxation:	None
Indicated monitors:	Standard
Postoperative analgesia:	I
Acceptable techniques:	GETA or heavy sedation

Comments: These patients may be children of any age with a wide range of congenital anomalies. (Or else why are you scanning them?) They may also be belligerent drunk motor vehicle accident victims from the ER or ICU. Your mission is to make the patient hold still for the scan in whatever way you can. A CT is less sensitive than an MRI but still requires stillness for each image.

Be wary of the patient who is "too sick to sedate": one with an intracranial mass and elevated intracranial pressure (ICP) who may become sedated all too easily. Sedation leads to respiratory depression, which leads to increased CO_2, which leads to an increase in ICP, which leads to more sedation, which leads to....Here in the northern hemisphere these patients will have a tendency to go down the drain clockwise.

CTs can often be accomplished with heavy sedation but will sometimes require a general anesthetic. Access to the patient will be difficult because the scanner is in the way, so you'll want to make sure you're happy with the anesthetic before allowing the scan to start (and removing yourself from the radiation-filled immediate vicinity). A continuous infusion of propofol or methohexital is better than repeated IV doses.

If you are scanning an intubated patient from the ICU or ER, make sure you contact respiratory therapy beforehand to arrange for a ventilator in the CT scan room. You will probably not want to bring your anesthesia machine there for a patient who can be easily managed with IV agents. Also be careful with patient transport; use a

monitor and supplemental oxygen if the patient is still sedated postprocedure.

Some scans require the injection of iodinated contrast material, which has a propensity for causing allergic reactions. Have the appropriate emergency drugs handy.

MRI Scan

Description: The patient is anesthetized, shifted to the gantry of the MRI scanner, secured in place with all appropriate monitoring, and the scan is begun. Your credit cards are simultaneously erased. That is all.

Position:	Supine, with airway 10 feet from anesthesia provider
Estimated time:	1 hour
Estimated blood loss:	Zero
Need for muscle relaxation:	None
Indicated monitors:	Standard
Postoperative analgesia:	I
Acceptable techniques:	GETA

Comments: Your patients will range from otherwise normal but claustrophobic adults all the way down to severely anomalous infants.

Your mission is to make the patient hold still, since even the slightest movement might wash out the whole study. An MRI will frequently require a general anesthetic, partly because of the length and noise of the procedure, partly because the patient will be 6 feet up the tube of the machine from you. Make sure that all of your anesthetic equipment and monitors are MRI-compatible. Check oxygen and nitrous hook-ups and the availability of suction equipment. Do all of this *before* the patient arrives.

Typically you will induce general anesthesia and intubate the patient on the stretcher, then move the patient to the gantry of the scanner. Make sure you have enough slack in your tubes and wires to reach all the way into the machine. Spontaneous ventilation is something to strive for, as it gives you one more monitor of anesthetic depth and allows patients to titrate their own anesthetic depth when you are using a volatile anesthetic. Your end-tidal CO_2 monitor will be sipping through a 20-foot hose, so it won't be quantitatively accurate. However, a wave form does indicate continued ventilation.

Anything metallic is a big problem for the MRI scanner. Loose metal, like laryngoscope blades, scissors, or stethoscopes, will fly toward the magnet, damaging it or anything that gets in the way. Metal attached to the patient—ECG leads, hip pins, surgical staples—may heat up and cause an injury.

Not only will your credit cards erase (and your pocket calculator, and your watch, and your beeper), but your monitors may also have trouble with the magnetic fields. Oximeters must be specially constructed to work with the MRI, and capnometer and blood pressure cables will have to extend out of the room to their base units (make sure you can see the numbers from wherever you end up standing). An ECG may be completely impossible, and you may just have to do without.

There's nothing harmful about staying in the scan room with the patient (as far as we know now), although it can be pretty loud. You're closer if anything happens, and you can keep a better eye on the patient's ventilation. Just make sure you can see all the monitors you have, and ask the technician to let you know when the end of the scan is approaching.

Gadolinium is given as an IV contrast agent for some studies. As far as we can tell, it has no effect on your anesthetic.

Know how to get at the patient's airway in a hurry. There's normally a manual override lever that lets you pull the patient out of the scanner, if you have to. Know where this is and how it works.

Transport from the MRI to the PACU can be an exciting adventure. Provide supplemental oxygen, use a transport monitor if the patient is not wide awake, and carry emergency drugs and airway equipment with you.

Neuroembolization

Description: In the angiography suite, the neuroradiologist identifies the blood supply to a tumor, arteriovenous malformation (AVM), or aneurysm, gets as close to it as possible with a catheter, and then injects it with some instantly coagulating compound. Sometimes this achieves a complete cure (as with AVMs). Other times it works to reduce bleeding at a subsequent definitive surgery. Sometimes it doesn't work at all. It always takes a long time.

Position:	Supine
Estimated time:	2 hours plus
Estimated blood loss:	Minimal
Need for muscle relaxation:	None
Indicated monitors:	Standard
Postoperative analgesia:	I
Acceptable techniques:	MAC, GETA

Comments: MAC is desirable because, on the one hand, the radiologist likes to have the patient awake enough to tell him if he suddenly strokes (it happens), and on the other hand, the radiologist likes to have the patient comfortable enough to tolerate the injections—which can cause a very painful burning sensation—without a lot of moving around. Your presence is especially constructive if the lesion being embolized is in a sensitive area and hemodynamic perturbations are anticipated.

General anesthesia may be necessary from the outset if the radiologist needs you to control the patient's ventilation so he can see what he's doing. This is common with lesions of the thoracic spine. More often, though, general anesthesia becomes a requirement after several hours of gradually deepening sedation. Make sure that before starting you have all the drugs and equipment (including your anesthesia machine) you will need when this happens.

Talk to the radiologist or the technicians to figure out how you can get to the patient's head in an emergency. If nothing else, it will let them know that an emergency is possible and that they'd better believe you if you say that you need to get to the patient.

Hemodynamic stimulation is impressive with intra-arterial injections but usually very short-lived. In potentially unstable patients you may want an arterial line and some vasoactive substances on hand to manage these crises. Esmolol, phenylephrine, and nitroprusside are all quite useful.

These cases can arise as emergencies. If you find yourself doing general anesthesia on a sick patient in the middle of the night four floors from your OR, make sure you know where your backup is and how long it'll take him or her to get to you.

Stereotactic Biopsy

Description: This procedure is done to obtain a tissue biopsy of an intracranial lesion seen on CT or MRI. The patient is first placed in a stereotactic frame, a circumferential device that fits over the face and head and is pinned to the patient's cranium. Then a scan is done to localize the lesion and provide coordinates for it relative to the frame. Then the patient is transported to the OR, where a burr hole is placed and a biopsy needle advanced to the exact spot indicated by the scan. Once the specimen is taken the procedure may be over or may go on to a craniotomy for excision.

Position:	Supine
Estimated time:	1 hour, not counting scan time
Estimated blood loss:	Minimal
Need for muscle relaxation:	None
Indicated monitors:	Standard
Postoperative analgesia:	II
Acceptable techniques:	MAC, GETA

Comments: Patients may be of any age or illness but are usually not too debilitated.

Cancer concerns apply (see Chapter 1).

Local anesthesia is generally used for placement of the pins that hold the stereotactic frame to the patient's head and for the scalp and periosteum of the skull. The brain itself lacks pain receptors.

Your role is to determine whether the patient can tolerate a MAC and to help him or her through the procedure. Access to the airway will be limited once the stereotactic frame is on, so the patient must be intubated before going to the scanner if you think that general anesthesia is indicated. Obviously, this is necessary if the surgeons are planning an excision based on the biopsy results. Alternatively, you might want to plan for an awake fiberoptic technique to secure the airway with the frame in place, if general anesthesia becomes necessary.

It's a good idea to look over the equipment before starting the case. Besides making sure that the frame is

MRI-compatible (if that's where you're headed) you can ascertain how to remove it in a hurry if necessary.

You might want to read the appropriate MRI or CT scan section above if you will be accompanying the patient through that portion of the procedure. Also see the introduction to Chapter 17.

Laminectomy/Discectomy

Description: The surgeon makes a vertical midline incision in the back and separates the muscle layers down to the spine. Various power tools are used to take off one or more laminae, decompressing the spinal canal and providing the surgeon access to the protruding portions of intervertebral disk, which are then ripped out with something from Daddy's toolbox. Depending on how much instability has been created, a bone graft may be placed between the laminae using either banked bone or a fresh piece nibbled off the iliac crest. Closure is usually fairly rapid.

Position:	Prone on one of several frames; rarely kneeling or lateral
Estimated time:	2 hours
Estimated blood loss:	200 ml; type and cross-match 2 units
Need for muscle relaxation:	Helpful, but see below*
Indicated monitors:	Standard
Postoperative analgesia:	II
Acceptable techniques:	GETA

Comments: Back surgery patients are usually fairly healthy but may have been playing the chronic pain game for a long time. Make sure they get their regular analgesics (excepting nonsteroidal anti-inflammatory drugs) up to the time of surgery, and plan a very gradual taper postoperatively. Local anesthetics injected into the wound during closure will help with analgesia.

The anesthesia usually begins supine on a stretcher, and the patient is then turned prone onto the operating table. That is a good time for IVs to come out and monitors to be lost, so pay close attention. The arms are either tucked at the sides or extended out and forward (the "Superman position"). In the latter case your antecubital

---

*Muscle relaxation is very reassuring for you, the anesthetist, because it reduces the chance that the patient will cough and buck and lose the endotracheal tube. No relaxation is comforting for the surgeon because he can count on something twitching if he bashes a nerve root. We usually try to keep the patient titrated to about one twitch on a train of four, which we hope will satisfy everyone.

IV will probably stop working, so don't put it there in the first place.

An operation in the prone position means you should secure your endotracheal tube very carefully. Be wary of your tape loosening as saliva soaks through it. You will also want to check the patient's positioning before letting the surgeon start the prep. Make sure that the face, ears, arms, breasts, genitals, and legs are all comfortably arranged and that all of your IV lines and monitors are still working.

Document all pre-existing neurologic deficits carefully.

Anesthetic alternatives include doing the case with a spinal or epidural (allowing the surgeon to provide a top-up dose if needed) or intubating the patient awake, nasally, and allowing the patient to position himself or herself on the table before inducing general anesthesia. A nasal intubation will secure the tube better than an oral approach. Both options help avoid some of the dangers of turning and positioning a patient under general anesthesia, but both will require careful preplanning and discussion with the patient and surgeon.

Don't wake the patient until you have turned him or her supine and checked all your monitors. Be wary of sudden blood pressure shifts with any change in position.

Anterior Cervical Disk (ACD)

Description: Through a diagonal incision in the lateral neck the surgeon will separate the muscle layers and expose the anterolateral disk space. The offending disk is removed from its contact with the nerve root, along with any bone that might be impinging, and a bone graft from a cadaver or from the patient's hip is used to shore up any weak spots. Plates and screws are used to stabilize the spine if necessary and the wound is closed.

Position:	Supine
Estimated time:	2 hours plus
Estimated blood loss:	100 ml; type and cross-match 2 units
Need for muscle relaxation:	Helpful; may be contraindicated
Indicated monitors:	Standard; consider Foley, SSEPs
Postoperative analgesia:	II
Acceptable techniques:	GETA

Comments: The patients are generally in fairly good health, with cervical disk disease that is limiting their normal functioning. In your preoperative assessment it is very important to determine what the patient's symptoms consist of (arm weakness, pain, paresthesia, etc.) and what his or her tolerance is for movement of the head and neck.

It is not uncommon for patients to have a severe enough limitation of mobility in the neck or sufficiently unstable anatomy to mandate an awake intubation with minimal movement. Once the tube is in and the patient is positioned for surgery, voluntary muscle function is tested before inducing anesthesia.

The surgeon may prefer the patient to not have complete neuromuscular blockade so that inadvertent dissection of a nerve or nerve root will manifest as patient movement.

Find out what the surgeon intends before starting the case. The patient for ACD with fusion and bone grafting will be in the OR for 4–5 hours, lose 200 ml of blood, and definitely need a Foley catheter. A simple

ACD, on the other hand, will be closer to the numbers shown above.

Wake the patient gently. Coughing or bucking may be detrimental to the surgical repair.

Anterolateral Craniotomy for Tumor

Description: After induction of anesthesia and positioning of the patient in pins, the surgeon lifts off a flap of bone over the area of interest, opens the dura, and separates the brain down to the site of the lesion. After carefully freeing it from the surrounding tissue, the surgeon removes the specimen, establishes hemostasis, closes the dura, closes the cranium, and closes the skin.

Position:	Supine or lateral decubitus, with airway away from you
Estimated time:	4 hours
Estimated blood loss:	300 ml; type and cross-match 2 units
Need for muscle relaxation:	Required
Indicated monitors:	Standard, 5-lead, Foley, A-line
Postoperative analgesia:	III
Acceptable techniques:	GETA, local in scalp is helpful

Comments: A wide variety of patient types present for craniotomy, from young and healthy to old and possessed of multiple medical problems. Those who are on phenytoin preoperatively will metabolize thiopental, narcotics, and some relaxants much faster than expected, so be prepared.

The typical anesthetic is designed to provide an absolutely immobile surgical field, yet allow prompt emergence and extubation at the end of the case. The neurosurgeon will wish to evaluate the patient's neurologic function immediately postop. One approach is to use a continuous narcotic infusion (like sufentanil, 0.125–0.33 µg/kg/hr) combined with a trace of isoflurane (as needed to maintain adequate hemodynamics). Periods of maximal stimulation for the patient are intubation, pinning, scalp incision, cranial opening, and emergence. The brain parenchyma itself is insensate, so that the lengthiest part of the operation requires the lowest levels of anesthesia. Neuromuscular blocking agents are mandated because of the potential damage that can occur if the patient tries to move while secured in the pins of the head holder.

Lowering the patient's ICP to slacken the dura for the surgeons may be required. Have mannitol, furosemide, and dexamethasone handy to give when asked. If a brisk diuresis results—as it should—be prepared to follow the patient's serum potassium. Too rapid a fall may lead to ECG abnormalities. Rapid changes in blood volume will also send you on a roller coaster ride with the patient's blood pressure. Be prepared to smooth out the hills and valleys pharmacologically if necessary.

Check an arterial blood gas (ABG) soon after intubation to give yourself some sense of what the gradient between your capnometer and the patient's real carbon dioxide might be. Then you can guide your hyperventilation appropriately when the surgeon asks for it.

You will also want one or two very good IVs, in case the surgeon gets into something that bleeds. Ask the surgeon which way the patient will be oriented so you can figure out which side of the bed you and your machine are going to wind up on, and plan where to put the IV and arterial line.

Phenylephrine is a good drug to have on hand for those little dips in blood pressure that sometimes occur. Lots of labetalol or even nitroglycerin or nitroprusside will be handy at the end of the case when you are struggling to keep the pressure down with the isoflurane off. Hypertension is bad after tumor surgery in the head because it increases the chance of the patient having a critical bleed into the empty tumor bed.

Posterior Fossa Craniotomy

Description: After the patient has been induced, pinned, and positioned, the surgeon opens the posterior fossa and accomplishes whatever intracranial business brought him or her there.

Position:	Sitting or lateral "park bench"
Estimated time:	5 hours
Estimated blood loss:	200 ml; type and cross-match 2 units
Need for muscle relaxation:	Required, but....
Indicated monitors:	Standard, 5-lead, Foley, A-line, CVP (long-line), precordial Doppler stethoscope
Postoperative analgesia:	III
Acceptable techniques:	GETA, local in scalp is helpful

Comments: Most of the comments in the section on anterior craniotomy also apply to this case, so read that one first. The following considerations are unique to posterior fossa surgery:

Surgery near the brainstem can produce some interesting hemodynamic effects like complete cessation of everything including heart rate. Our usual response is "Hey! Stop that!" followed by atropine (for the patient) and nitroglycerin (for us). Generally asystole will resolve if the surgeon stops pushing on the brainstem, allowing time for the atropine to work and make the patient less sensitive to the effect before the surgeon goes back to work. In an analogous situation to spinal cord surgery the patient can also have postoperative cranial nerve deficits; make sure the patient can gag, cough, and swallow before extubating.

Acoustic neuromas are a common target of posterior fossa craniotomies. These can also be excised in a translabyrinthine approach by the ENT surgeons (see Chapter 3). Depending on the exact location of the tumor the surgeon may request brainstem auditory evoked responses (BAERs), which require special training to set up and interpret, or facial nerve motor function monitoring, which is relatively self-evident but requires that you keep the neuromuscular blockade to a minimum.

The greatest additional concern caused by surgery in the sitting position is the possibility of venous air embolism (VAE). The chance for VAE is increased in any situation in which there is a communication between the atmosphere and the venous system—as from an open bone or dural sinus—and a negative pressure gradient tending to draw air into the body. In craniotomies you will be trying to keep the patient very dry so that elevating the head above the heart may well create a negative CVP in the brain even in the presence of positive pressure ventilation.

VAE can be detected by (in order of decreasing sensitivity): transesophageal echocardiography (TEE), precordial Doppler, increased pulmonary artery pressure, suddenly decreased end-tidal CO_2, the presence of exhaled nitrogen, decreased oxygen saturation, decreased mean arterial pressure, and the characteristic "mill wheel" murmur.

Management of VAE consists of the following:

1. Giving 100% oxygen (both for support and because eliminating N_2O will decrease bubble size)
2. Stopping the inflow of air by flooding the surgical field with saline
3. Plugging bone with bone wax
4. Cauterizing or oversewing the dura
5. Positioning the patient with the head down (use the Trendelenburg handle) and the right side up (keeping the air away from the right ventricular outflow tract)
6. Aspiration of air from a catheter in the right atrium (positioned preoperatively by x-ray or ECG signal)
7. Providing whatever hemodynamic support is needed including CPR

Factors that influence the outcome from an episode of VAE are the volume of gas embolized, the time course over which the embolization occurs, the presence of a patent foramen ovale (found in up to 30% of adults), the use of nitrous oxide, and the patient's baseline myocardial function.

Craniotomy for Aneurysm Clipping

Description: After induction, intubation, pinning, and positioning, the neurosurgeon gently dissects down to the aneurysm and puts a metal clip on it to remove it from the circulation. Then he closes. Sounds easy, doesn't it?

Position:	Depends on location of aneurysm
Estimated time:	4 hours
Estimated blood loss:	200 ml plus; type and crossmatch 6 units
Need for muscle relaxation:	Required
Indicated monitors:	Standard, 5-lead, Foley, A-line; consider SSEP or EEG
Postoperative analgesia:	III
Acceptable techniques:	GETA, local in the scalp is helpful

Comments: Intracranial aneurysms occur in 20% of the population, but obviously most of these are asymptomatic. Subarachnoid hemorrhage from an aneurysm is a medical emergency that requires prompt intervention to prevent rebleeding.

Many of the considerations for this case are the same as for anterior or posterior fossa craniotomies, so don't forget to read those sections. Also look at the ICP considerations at the start of this chapter.

Your preoperative evaluation should focus on the location and size of the aneurysm and the symptoms it has caused the patient. You are unlikely to extubate the patient at the end of the case if the mental status was impaired preoperatively, no matter how successful the surgery. Neurologic deficits may consist of mass effects, focal findings, or global impairment caused by increased ICP. ECG abnormalities are common, and may not correlate with myocardial ischemia. Similarly, myocardial dysfunction and pulmonary edema can occur in the absence of ischemia or ECG changes.

Patient preparation should include two large IVs and an arterial line. Consider a CVP from the arm or subclavian (in the internal jugular it may impede venous out-flow from the brain, thereby raising ICP).

Aneurysms that have bled once are at high risk for rebleeding, so careful control of the blood pressure is essential. The guiding principle for anesthetizing a patient with a cerebral aneurysm should be to maintain the "transmural pressure gradient" to minimize the risk of rupture. Generous sedation during painful procedures is one approach but can lead to respiratory depression and increased ICP; changes in mental status also become difficult to determine in the sedated patient. The best answer is to sedate lightly and not futz around.

Intraoperatively your goals are to prevent rapid changes in blood pressure or ICP that can precipitate rebleeding, to decrease the brain's metabolic rate, to maintain cerebral blood flow, to facilitate the surgeon's dissection by shrinking the brain at the right moment, and to wake up the patient on a dime at the end of the case so that subsequent neurologic changes can be promptly noted.

Be prepared to lower the patient's blood pressure precipitously when the surgeon requests it. Decreased blood pressure will shrink the aneurysm and decrease its likelihood of rupturing as the surgeon closes in on it. Nitroprusside or isoflurane can be used, but beware of lowering the pressure to the point where normal brain is becoming ischemic. Barbiturate coma or near-coma ("burst suppression"), guided by EEG monitoring, may be used to decrease $CMRO_2$ and provide a wider margin of safety during induced hypotension or temporary clip placement.

Vasospasm does not usually occur until 48 hours after a subarachnoid hemorrhage—after the aneurysm has been surgically dealt with, we hope. Symptoms may range from nothing all the way up to massive stroke and global neurologic deficit. Treatment consists of the "triple H": making the patient *h*ypervolemic, *h*ypertensive, and *h*yperdynamic, usually guided by a pulmonary artery catheter to determine just how hard the patient's heart can be pushed. Needless to say, if the aneurysm has not yet been dealt with, hypertension may not be a good idea.

Transsphenoidal Hypophysectomy

Description: The surgeon makes a small incision under the upper lip and dissects up through the nasal septum and sphenoid sinus to the pituitary fossa, where he or she removes the offending tumor. The holes are plugged, the incisions are closed, and off you go to the PACU.

Position:	Supine with the head up or sitting "beach chair"
Estimated time:	4 hours
Estimated blood loss:	100 ml; type and cross-match 2 units
Need for muscle relaxation:	Required
Indicated monitors:	Standard, 5-lead, Foley, A-line
Postoperative analgesia:	II
Acceptable techniques:	GETA

Comments: This operation is the method of choice for the resection of pituitary tumors that do not have extensive suprasellar involvement. For patients with suprasellar extension or with optic nerve involvement, a transcranial approach is usually preferred.

Pituitary adenomas come in a variety of flavors. Prolactinomas and tumors that secrete thyroid-stimulating hormone, follicle-stimulating hormone, and luteinizing hormone cause no extra problems. Tumors that secrete adrenocorticotropic hormone cause Cushing's disease: hyperaldosteronism, decreased potassium, metabolic alkalosis, hypertension, congestive heart failure (CHF), and truncal obesity. IV access will be difficult, and the patient will ultimately require steroid supplementation, although not on your time. Growth hormone–secreting tumors may cause gigantism, acromegaly, hypertension, cardiomegaly, CHF, and severe anatomic airway abnormalities, including glottic stenosis. Be prepared for trouble with these patients.

Increased ICP is not usually a concern with these patients. Your anesthetic goals are to provide the surgeon with an immobile field, a hemodynamically stable patient, and a quick wake-up at the end of the case. We usually achieve this with some sort of narcotic infusion and generous neuromuscular blockade.

An oral endotracheal tube is required. The surgeon will probably place a throat pack in the pharynx to absorb blood dripping down from the nose; make sure it comes out at the end of the case.

The surgeon may place cocaine pledgets in the nares and/or inject the mucosa with epinephrine-containing local anesthetics. This decreases bleeding and benefits your anesthetic, although inadvertent intravascular injections may cause hypertension, tachycardia, or dysrhythmias.

The pituitary gland is located in the sella turcica, the lateral walls of which are composed of a thin layer of bone over a large layer of cavernous sinus. Wandering into this territory can get you into trouble with cranial nerves III–VI, the carotid artery (which bleeds), the cavernous sinus, and the whole venous air embolism thing. (See the section on posterior fossa for guidance on VAE.)

The patient's nose will be occluded with gauze packs at the end of the procedure, so he or she must be wide awake and able to breathe comfortably through the mouth before extubation. Thorough suctioning is essential, as stray blood in the airway is a strong stimulus for laryngospasm.

Cranial Decompression (Burr Holes)

Description: The surgeon makes a small scalp incision, then drills a hole through the cranium and opens the dura underneath. Accumulated blood can be removed through the hole and/or a ventriculostomy can be placed to monitor and adjust CSF pressure.

Position:	Supine, head elevated to reduce ICP
Estimated time:	1 hour
Estimated blood loss:	Minimal; type and cross-match 2 units
Need for muscle relaxation:	Helpful
Indicated monitors:	Standard; consider A-line
Postoperative analgesia:	II
Acceptable techniques:	GETA, local

Comments: Burr holes are placed to relieve elevated ICP either by removing an epidural or subdural hematoma or by allowing the placement of a ventriculostomy. Symptomatic elevation of ICP is an emergency situation usually caused by trauma but occasionally by bleeding from a tumor or aneurysm. This case will crash in on you when you least expect it.

Patients with stable hematomas and depressed mental status (as is common after a motor vehicle accident, for instance) may have their burr holes placed in the ICU or ER. Patients who are unstable, capable of perceiving painful stimuli, or likely to progress to a craniotomy will come to you in the OR. Your job is to secure the airway, support the patient, and let the neurosurgeon get going as soon as possible.

Playing the ICP game during induction and intubation is essential. See this chapter's introduction for details. Drugs that blunt a hyperdynamic response, like narcotics or IV lidocaine, are your best friends.

Most of these patients will have full stomachs. Succinylcholine allows for a rapid intubation but may transiently increase ICP. High-dose vecuronium may be a better choice. Don't forget the cricoid pressure.

Hyperventilate the patient before, during, and after induction. Other than keeping the head up it's the easiest and quickest way to lower ICP.

Distal Nerve Surgery

Description: The surgeon opens the skin over the entrapped nerve, frees it up from any constricting tissue or reroutes it by a shorter route around a bone, and closes.

Position:	Supine
Estimated time:	2 hours
Estimated blood loss:	Minimal; type and screen
Need for muscle relaxation:	Contraindicated
Indicated monitors:	Standard, intraoperative electromyography (EMG)
Postoperative analgesia:	II
Acceptable techniques:	GA, MAC

Comments: This procedure is done to relieve an entrapped nerve, most typically the ulnar nerve at the elbow. The patients are usually young and otherwise healthy.

Regional anesthesia will complicate postoperative assessment of the involved nerve and is therefore usually avoided.

Muscle relaxation may make it hard for the surgeon to detect damage to the nerve as it is freed from the surrounding tissue, as well as interfering with EMG monitoring, and is therefore usually avoided.

Another distal nerve procedure that you may encounter is the sural nerve biopsy. This relatively useless nerve is occasionally sacrificed in an effort to find a diagnosis for patients with obscure neuromuscular diseases. The operation is done in the prone position and is usually short. Blood loss is minimal. Any anesthetic technique is acceptable although the surgeon may elect to do the procedure under local alone. Since the patient has an uncharacterized neuromuscular disorder you'll probably be just as happy to be uninvolved.

Cranioplasty

Description: The surgeon makes a scalp incision over the area of concern, removes any excess bone, and fashions a plastic or bone-banked replacement for any missing section. The new piece is secured with wires and the scalp is closed.

Position:	Depends on location of defect
Estimated time:	2 hours
Estimated blood loss:	100 ml; type and cross-match 2 units
Need for muscle relaxation:	Not required
Indicated monitors:	Standard; consider Foley
Postoperative analgesia:	II; local in scalp will help with analgesia
Acceptable techniques:	GETA

Comments: This operation is done to fix a defect in the bones of the skull, either congenital or related to a previous neurosurgery. The procedure is essentially a cosmetic one and will be entirely extradural.

The scalp tends to bleed generously, but this problem can be diminished with pre-emptive injection of a local anesthetic solution with epinephrine.

As with almost all neurosurgeries, it is important to secure your endotracheal tube well since you won't have good access to it during the case.

Venous air embolism is a possibility if the patient is in the sitting position and large venous sinuses in the area are exposed. Read about this complication in the section on posterior fossa craniotomy and urge the surgeons to use plenty of bone wax.

In pediatric patients a cranioplasty usually means the correction of a craniosynostosis, a congenital defect in skull formation. The operation is about the same as in adults except that in a neonate a 100-ml blood loss may represent half the patient's blood volume. Talk with the surgeon before you start one of these and find out how big a deal it's going to be, then read our chapter on pediatric surgery for some general pointers.

Ventriculoperitoneal (V-P) Shunt

Description: The surgeon makes a burr hole in the head and introduces a ventriculostomy catheter. The catheter is then connected to a long plastic tube that is tunneled subcutaneously down to the abdomen and secured in the peritoneum. A one-way valve ensures that fluid will only flow from the brain to the belly and not the other way around.

Position:	Supine, head turned to the side
Estimated time:	2 hours
Estimated blood loss:	Minimal; type and screen
Need for muscle relaxation:	Helpful
Indicated monitors:	Standard
Postoperative analgesia:	II
Acceptable techniques:	GETA

Comments: This procedure is commonly done on children with some form of hydrocephalus to relieve the swelling in the brain and allow them to maintain a normal ICP. Needless to say, children grow over time, and it is not unusual to have to go back years later and revise (lengthen) the shunt.

Children with hydrocephalus commonly have other anomalies. Take a good look at the airway and a good listen to the heart before inducing anesthesia.

Sterile technique is important in handling the child since an infected shunt is a major problem.

And another thing about kids: the prep will extend from the head to the belly, usually on the right side, creating a large surface area for heat loss. The right arm will be tucked so the left side is usually better for lines and monitors.

Tape your tube carefully, since manipulation of the head is often necessary in the pediatric patient. Inadvertent extubation is not at all uncommon.

Spinal Rodding

Description: The surgeon makes a long, vertical mid-line incision over the unstable or scoliotic region of the spine, exposes all the laminae on both sides, fastens hardware to various points above, below, and throughout the area of interest, and then puts in a couple of vertical rods to provide support and allow weight-bearing.

Position:	Prone
Estimated time:	8 hours
Estimated blood loss:	1,000 ml plus; type and crossmatch 6 units
Need for muscle relaxation:	Contraindicated
Indicated monitors:	Standard, Foley, A-line, SSEP; consider CVP/PA line
Postoperative analgesia:	III
Acceptable techniques:	GETA

Comments: This case is a real lulu! Expect a lot of bleeding, a lot of heat loss, and a big third-space fluid loss. Plan to have plenty of IV access, and keep the patient warm from the start.

Associated disease states with scoliosis include restrictive lung disease, malignant hyperthermia, airway anomalies, neurologic deficits, and neuromuscular disorders such as muscular dystrophy.

For any surgery in the prone position, make sure the endotracheal tube is well secured and that all of the patient's pressure points are well padded. If the arms are tucked at the sides, make sure all the lines and monitors are working before allowing the surgeons to start the prep.

One of the big questions with scoliosis surgery is whether the surgeon has distracted (straightened) the spinal cord enough or too much. There are two common approaches for assessing neurologic function intra-op: somatosensory evoked potentials (SSEPs) and the wake-up test.

SSEPs measure the brainstem response to a stimulus provided at a distal sensory nerve, typically the posterior tibial. If the spinal cord gets stretched and ischemic the SSEP signal will change (typically decreased amplitude and increased latency) and you will be able to tell the surgeon that a problem exists. Setting up and interpreting an SSEP requires a well-trained technician.

The wake-up test is just that and is intended to measure motor function. It is therefore complementary with the SSEPs, rather than redundant, and you may be asked to do both. When the surgeon has finished straightening out the cord, you will be asked to awaken the patient enough to find out if the toes still wiggle on command. There are a lot of anesthetic recipes available for doing this, but we like an approach involving a narcotic infusion, a minimum of volatile anesthetic, and a relaxant. When wake-up time approaches, the volatile anesthetic is turned off, the relaxant is allowed to resolve, and the patient is interrogated. With luck (and the right dose of narcotics) the patient will follow the commands you give without a whole lot of unsightly coughing or bucking. It's a good idea to warn the patient about the test before starting the case, since he or she will have a fair chance of remembering it later. It's also a good idea not to use neuromuscular reversal agents or naloxone since you are going to want to put the patient immediately back to sleep once the test is completed.

Spinal Cord Tumor Resection

Description: The surgeon opens the spine over the tumor and resects it with as large a margin as possible while preserving as many nerves as possible. Hemostasis is then achieved and the remaining tissue defect assessed. Bone graft, plates, and even spinal rods may be necessary to restore spinal stability.

Position:	Depends on the location of the tumor
Estimated time:	All day
Estimated blood loss:	2,000 ml plus; type and crossmatch 8 units
Need for muscle relaxation:	See below
Indicated monitors:	Standard, Foley, A-line, SSEP; consider CVP or PA line
Postoperative analgesia:	III or IV
Acceptable techniques:	GETA

Comments: This case is a big deal and will consume an immense amount of OR resources. The neurosurgeon may need help from the thoracic, general, orthopedic, or ENT services in approaching the tumor, depending on where it's located. You should prepare yourself for a long day.

The patient may be young and otherwise healthy (primary bone or nervous tissue tumors) or old and debilitated (metastases from breast, colon, prostate, lung, etc.). Operations in the former group tend to be planned and coordinated weeks in advance; operations in the latter group tend to be much more ad hoc, and are often done on an emergent basis.

Blood loss will be the theme for the day. Prepare yourself by obtaining lots of large-bore IV access, ideally in areas that will not interfere with the surgical procedure or patient positioning. Warn the blood bank that you may need their help; get yourself a heated rapid infuser, and start transfusing as soon as things start to look bad. Bleeding can be quite brisk from bony cancers and very hard to control. One thing that may save you, which you should ask the surgeon about, is a neuroembolization by the radiologist prior to starting the surgery.

A second theme will be assessment of neurologic function. SSEPs are useful as a continuous monitor but require expert application and interpretation. Keeping the patient unparalyzed can be beneficial while the surgeon is working near the spinal cord.

Even though the surgeon will be hot to talk to the patient postoperatively to determine what's working and what's not, you should not plan to wake up the patient if you've had to give a lot of blood and fluid. Let the patient warm up, diurese, and clear all the anesthesia before extubating.

Thoracic Surgery

Welcome to thoracic surgery, where you get to learn about breathing!

You may have thought you had this skill mastered early in life, but that was not, in fact, the case. You haven't really breathed until you've done it on one lung through a tracheostomy while having pulmonary hypertension. Or how about ventilating the left lung with a 5.0 endotracheal tube by hand while ventilating the right lung through a sawed-off suction catheter attached to a high-frequency jet while the surgeon takes out the carina in between. Now that's breathing!

In thoracic anesthesia you learn to establish and manage patients on one-lung ventilation while the other lung is being operated on.

Besides learning how to handle the complex airway while the surgeons are working on it, you will also learn about managing roller coaster anesthetics. Stimulation from a rigid bronchoscopy, for example, can be excruciating one second and completely gone the next. Even with a thoracic epidural dosed to the gills, a thoracotomy patient can respond impressively when the surgeons tug on the carina (which is innervated by the vagus nerve, arising above the gills). And don't think you're going to smooth things out with a bunch of narcotics either! That technique is for those weenie anesthesiologists who work on the spacer. (You know, that organ that holds the lungs apart.) Here on the thoracic service we expect your patient to wake up and breathe well on his or her own, as soon as the case is finished.

Thoracic patients are fortunately less bothered by swings in blood pressure than cardiac patients. Patients with both bad hearts and bad lungs usually don't make it to the OR, so you can worry less about ejection fraction and ischemic threshold and more about pulmonary function tests (PFTs), split function lung studies, and room air arterial blood gases (ABGs).

In the technical arena you will prosper on the thoracic service, picking up plenty of arterial lines, endobronchial intubations, thoracic epidurals, and flexible bronchoscopies.

Rigid Bronchoscopy

Description: The surgeon sticks a straight steel tube through the vocal cords and down the trachea. A telescope with a 0-, 30-, or 60-degree angle on the tip goes through the tube to allow the surgeon to look around in the proximal bronchi. Devices exist for suctioning, taking biopsies, and cauterizing through the rigid bronchoscope.

Position:	Supine, head dropped back, shoulders raised, arms tucked
Estimated time:	30 minutes
Estimated blood loss:	Zero
Need for muscle relaxation:	Very helpful
Indicated monitors:	Standard
Postoperative analgesia:	I
Acceptable techniques:	GETA

Comments: This procedure is typically done on patients with tracheal lesions and may be merely the prelude to an attempted resection. Patients with tracheal papillomas may have repeated rigid bronchoscopies for laser or conventional excision. Because of the interference with vocal cord function and the lack of a tracheal seal, aspiration prophylaxis is recommended in all these patients.

Ventilation must occur through the bronchoscope. Following induction and establishment of a deep level of anesthesia via the face mask, the surgeon places the bronchoscope through the cords and ventilation is reestablished using either a jet injector or a side port.

Jet ventilation works through an open scope by entraining room air with a high-flow jet of pure oxygen. The jet must be pointed straight down the trachea to provide adequate ventilation, which can be assessed by chest rise, oximetry, and ABGs. FiO_2 and end-tidal gas monitoring are not possible using the jet, and a totally IV anesthetic technique must be used.

Side port bronchoscopes have a built-in connection for the anesthesia circuit and are designed to be used with a glass stopper at the proximal end. Volatile anesthesia can be used (with a variable amount of leak), although ventilation by hand is required since compliance will change with movement of the scope and since the eye-piece will be periodically removed to allow suctioning or instrumentation.

Make sure the surgeon places a tooth guard over the upper incisors.

Muscle relaxation is a good idea because the procedure can be intermittently very stimulating and the consequences of coughing are severe.

If a laser is going to be involved make sure you read the appropriate section in Chapter 1, as well as the following procedure description.

Laser Excision of Tracheal Lesion

Description: Through a rigid bronchoscope, an operating laryngoscope, or an endotracheal tube the surgeon lines up the target tissue with the laser guide and fires away.

Position:	Supine, head back, shoulders raised, arms tucked
Estimated time:	60 minutes
Estimated blood loss:	Minimal
Need for muscle relaxation:	Very helpful
Indicated monitors:	Standard
Postoperative analgesia:	I
Acceptable techniques:	GETA

Comments: Lasering a tracheal lesion has the advantage of immediately cauterizing the underlying tissue, and the technique is therefore slowly gaining in popularity. Besides, the disadvantages are mostly experienced by the anesthesiologist, not the surgeon.

Igniting an endotracheal tube with a laser is a very real and very scary prospect. For this reason you should use a special tube that has been manufactured or prepared to be fire resistant. Fill the cuff with saline instead of air (some would even go so far as to add methylene blue, so as to know when the cuff is ruptured). Maintain as low an FiO_2 as possible to reduce the chance of a fire, and avoid the use of nitrous oxide, which also supports combustion. Keep a source of irrigating fluid on hand to douse the trachea. And—most important—**pull the tube out if a fire occurs!**

Keep the patient paralyzed and deeply anesthetized when the lasering is going on, but be warned that the procedure can finish quite suddenly. Use drugs that are easy to get rid of.

Think for a moment about the potential for edema or bleeding at the surgical site before extubating the patient. Reintubation can be incredibly difficult if the airway is already compromised.

See the section on lasers in Chapter 1 for more information.

Rigid Esophagoscopy

Description: The surgeon sticks a long steel tube down the patient's throat, potentially all the way to the gastroesophageal junction, and looks around. There are a variety of grabbing, biting, and snipping instruments that can be used to take biopsies or resect tissue through the tube.

Position:	Supine, head back
Estimated time:	30 minutes
Estimated blood loss:	Zero
Need for muscle relaxation:	Helpful
Indicated monitors:	Standard
Postoperative analgesia:	I
Acceptable techniques:	GETA

Comments: Typically done either as the first step in an esophageal resection (to define the location of the lesion) or to relieve a strictured esophagus. In the latter circumstance the same patient may present for esophagoscopy dozens of times over many years. The typical rigid esophagoscopy patient should be considered to have a full stomach.

Flexible esophagoscopy is covered in the section on upper endoscopy in Chapter 2. A flexible 'scoping is relatively benign and can be accomplished under topical anesthesia. Rigid esophagoscopy is enormously stimulating and requires a general anesthetic.

Use of a smaller than normal endotracheal tube with less air in the cuff will allow the surgeon more room to work behind the trachea. Use of a tooth guard (like a boxer's mouthpiece) will help protect the upper incisors from abuse by the scope.

Since the complications of rigid esophagoscopy mostly relate to inadvertent perforation—pneumothorax, pneumomediastinum, bleeding, cardiac tamponade, dysrhythmias, mediastinal or pleural infection—the use of muscle relaxants to keep the patient still is probably a good idea.

The procedure ends abruptly. Consider using general anesthetics like propofol or desflurane that are easy to turn off when you want the patient to wake up.

Tracheostomy

Description: The surgeon cuts a hole in the neck, finds the trachea, opens the anterior surface in one way or another, asks you to pull back your tube, and stuffs in his own. Ventilation is switched over to the tracheostomy tube, which is then secured as the neck wound is closed.

Position:	Supine, shoulders raised, head extended back, arms tucked
Estimated time:	45 minutes
Estimated blood loss:	Minimal
Need for muscle relaxation:	Helpful
Indicated monitors:	Standard, plus whatever the patient already has
Postoperative analgesia:	I
Acceptable techniques:	GETA, local

Comments: Typically performed on critically ill patients where a long course on a ventilator is anticipated (or already under way). These patients may be extremely sick and may come to you on multiple vasoactive infusions. Indeed, transporting the tracheostomy patient to and from the ICU may be more time-consuming and difficult than the case itself. You will want to travel each way with everything you might need to reintubate the patient, as well as a fistful of useful drugs.

Rarely, a tracheostomy will even be done in the ICU. Most places are not set up for this, though, and will resist the temptation unless the patient is extremely unstable.

General anesthesia may be established with a large dose of fentanyl, nitrous oxide, and a relaxant. The patient is put on 100% oxygen before the tracheostomy is actually placed. Relaxants will help keep the patient from bucking during the procedure (which is only intermittently stimulating) and may help to keep lines in during transport but will make it impossible for the patient to breathe spontaneously if the airway is lost.

When you back up the endotracheal tube, try not to remove it all the way. Every so often the surgeon will have a problem with the tracheostomy and will want you to readvance your tube. Close communication is important.

Local anesthesia can be used for tracheostomies in patients who are not already intubated and have scary-looking airways. The ENT surgeons are especially good at this. When instrumenting an existing tracheostomy, a spray of topical anesthesia will help keep the patient from responding.

Do not mess with a recent tracheostomy. Any adjustments that need to be made in the first 24–48 hours should be referred to the surgeons, as a dislodged tube in a patient whose tracheostomy has not yet "matured" may be very hard to replace. If you are ever confronted with an accidental decannulation, remember that the easiest way to fix it is with a laryngoscope and an endotracheal tube from above.

Mediastinoscopy

Description: Through a small incision just above the sternum the surgeon dissects bluntly down into the anterior mediastinum, using an instrument a lot like an operating laryngoscope to lift up the sternum and illuminate the space beneath. Various instruments exist for taking biopsies and cauterizing tissue at the bottom of the deep dark hole.

Position:	Supine, head back, shoulders bumped up, arms tucked
Estimated time:	60 minutes
Estimated blood loss:	Minimal plus
Need for muscle relaxation:	Helpful
Indicated monitors:	Standard, A-line
Postoperative analgesia:	II
Acceptable techniques:	GETA

Comments: This procedure may be done specifically to obtain tissue, as in the young patient with a lymphoma, or to exclude mediastinal involvement of a lung cancer before carrying on with a resection.

Paralysis is helpful to avoid patient movement during the delicate parts of the procedure. This operation is minimally stimulating until the surgeon whacks the trachea, at which point the patient will try to get up and leave if not adequately anesthetized.

An arterial line or oximeter on the left side will provide an uninterrupted signal. On the right side, interruptions in flow will be periodically evident as the innominate artery becomes compressed between the mediastinoscope and the underside of the sternum. We usually put one monitor on each hand so we always know what's going on. Some authorities recommend a second IV line in the patient's foot for dealing with compression or damage to the superior vena cava.

And on that subject—the most interesting thing about mediastinoscopies is their potential to go dramatically bad. If the surgeon biopsies the bronchus, pulmonary artery or vein, azygos vein, vena cava, innominate artery, or heart, the resulting complication will be talked about in your department for years to come. And you'll wish you had a large-bore IV.

If the mediastinoscopy is to be followed immediately by a thoracoscopy or thoracotomy, expect a wait at the end of the procedure while your pathologist looks over the frozen sections. Depending on how things work at your hospital, you may be able to use this time to close the mediastinoscopy wound, put in a double-lumen tube, and position for a thoracotomy. Or you may just want to wait.

Thoracoscopy

Description: A small incision is made over the rib, and an entry port is punched into the pleural space. A thoracoscope connected to a camera is inserted. Once the lung has been allowed to collapse, the surgeon is able to get quite a good view of the chest cavity. Additional ports can be placed for manipulation of the lung or pleura up to and including staple resections of modest portions of lung tissue.

Position:	Lateral decubitus, arms extended anteriorly
Estimated time:	60 minutes plus
Estimated blood loss:	Minimal
Need for muscle relaxation:	Required
Indicated monitors:	Standard, A-line, Foley
Postoperative analgesia:	III
Acceptable techniques:	GETA, combined

Comments: This brand-new procedure is gaining popularity very rapidly since it spares the patient (and the surgeon) a long and painful incision accompanied by a long and painful recovery. It can make the case much longer, though, especially on those days when you do a thoracoscopy, cut out a wedge of lung, send it to pathology, get back a nasty cancer, and proceed on to a full thoracotomy.

In general, the number of thoracoscopies that become thoracotomies will depend on the patient's disease, the planned procedure, and the experience of the surgeon. If there's a reasonable chance that the procedure will become an open one, you should plan for the worst and place an arterial line and an epidural catheter preoperatively. An epidural may be useful for analgesia even if the chest remains closed.

One-lung ventilation (via double-lumen tube, bronchial blocker, or Univent) will be required for the procedure. Left-sided tubes are easier to position correctly and will function for either left- or right-sided thoracoscopies. The use of such a large tube and the potential difficulties involved with placing it correctly make preoperative aspiration prophylaxis prudent. Plan to use 100% oxygen during the times the lung is deflated.

This case can end quickly, since there may not be much incision to close. If any lung has been resected the surgeon will leave a chest tube in place, adding significantly to the patient's postoperative pain.

Extubating the patient while still in the decubitus position works surprisingly well and can speed your departure from the OR. Secretions will drain out the patient's mouth rather than onto the sensitive regions of the pharynx, and laryngospasm is very seldom encountered. Should reintubation be necessary, it is relatively easy to flop the patient back supine either on the OR bed or the gurney.

Pulmonary Lobe or Wedge Resection

Description: The chest is opened through a mini- or full-lateral thoracotomy, the diseased portion of lung is identified and dissected free, and a stapler is used to free the specimen. A chest tube is placed, and the wound is closed in multiple layers.

Position:	Lateral decubitus, arms extended anteriorly
Estimated time:	2 hours
Estimated blood loss:	200 ml; type and cross-match 2 units
Need for muscle relaxation:	Required
Indicated monitors:	Standard, Foley, A-line
Postoperative analgesia:	IV
Acceptable techniques:	GETA, combined

Comments: The arterial line and IV will be easier to manage and less likely to kink if they are placed in the dependent arm (the side opposite the surgery).

A double-lumen tube will be required for exposure. Most simple resections on either side can be done with a left-sided tube, which is easier to place correctly. The only indication for a right-sided tube (other than training, of course) is a left upper lobectomy that may become a left pneumonectomy. Use 100% oxygen and hand ventilation when clamping one lung off.

Large tubes and careful intubations make aspiration prophylaxis a good idea.

The pain after a thoracotomy is quite severe due to the multiple muscle layers involved and their continued postoperative stimulation by breathing and coughing. Respiratory function is clearly better postop with an epidural, although pain can also be controlled with intravenous patient-controlled anesthesia.

The surgeon may desire a pressure test of the suture/staple line at the end of the resection. After the chest cavity has been filled with saline, the operative lung is first gently suctioned free of blood and pooled secretions and then gradually reinflated to a pressure of 30–35 mm Hg. The resection line is inspected for air bubbles, and any gross air leaks are repaired.

Pulmonary resections are occasionally done through a median sternotomy incision. This is a little bit harder for the surgeon but leads to a quicker return of normal pulmonary function postoperatively. This approach is therefore used for patients with very marginal lung function or for those requiring bilateral wedge resections (typically young patients with metastatic osteosarcomas).

Extubating the patient on his or her side will generally work well since secretions will drain naturally out of the side of the mouth and will get you out of the OR faster. If you're leaving for an ICU, make sure you have oxygen and a transport monitor with you as well as drugs and equipment for emergency reintubation.

Pneumonectomy

Description: Through a posterolateral thoracotomy the entire lung is dissected clear of the pleura, the great vessels are ligated, and the lung is removed.

Position:	Lateral decubitus, arms extended anteriorly
Estimated time:	3 hours
Estimated blood loss:	500 ml; type and cross-match 2 units
Need for muscle relaxation:	Required
Indicated monitors:	Standard, Foley, A-line
Postoperative analgesia:	IV
Acceptable techniques:	GETA, combined

Comments: This operation is typically done for the patient with a lung cancer invading the hilar structures or the proximal bronchi. Preoperative assessment of lung function, including PFTs and split function studies, is important in determining if the patient can tolerate the loss of half or more of the pulmonary surface.

In general the procedure is similar to any other pulmonary resection (read the section on pulmonary lobe or wedge resection for details), but there are a few specific wrinkles.

A right-sided double-lumen tube may be required for left pneumonectomies. Sometimes the surgeon will be able to transect the bronchus below the end of a left-sided tube, but most times things will be easier with the tube on the right.

The surgeon will leave a chest tube (not on suction!) in place for 24 hours to serve as a drain for blood. Beyond this time period it becomes a potential conduit for infection of the empty chest cavity (which will eventually fill with serosanguinous fluid and scar down) and should therefore be removed.

Right pneumonectomies have a significantly higher mortality than left, due either to the larger amount of lung tissue removed or to interruption of the normal lymphatic drainage from the remaining left lung. The remaining lung is prone to developing adult respiratory distress syndrome (ARDS) postoperatively, which will be very poorly tolerated. You will want to keep the patient as far on the dry side as possible to minimize this possibility.

A rare postoperative complication of right pneumonectomies is herniation of the heart through the pericardial opening into the right chest cavity, kinking the great vessels and causing instantaneous death. This typically occurs when the patient is turned right side down (which might be attempted to improve ventilation in the remaining lung). If you see this happen, turn the patient back quickly, start CPR, and pray.

Pleural Stripping/Pleurodesis

Description: The pleura is approached through a lateral thoracotomy. If a resection is planned, the surgeon will laboriously peel the thickened pleura off the lung tissue using a combination of blunt and sharp dissection. Pleurodesis, on the other hand, simply involves roughing up the pleural surface with a cotton gauze, filling the pleural space with a fibrogenic agent like talcum powder, and closing. Pleurodesis is now commonly done through a thoracoscope.

Position:	Lateral decubitus, arms extended anteriorly
Estimated time:	1 hour for pleurodesis, 3 hours for pleural stripping
Estimated blood loss:	Minimal for pleurodesis, 700 ml for stripping; type and crossmatch 2 units
Need for muscle relaxation:	Required
Indicated monitors:	Standard, A-line, Foley
Postoperative analgesia:	IV
Acceptable techniques:	GETA, combined

Comments: Pleural stripping (as for a mesothelioma) takes a long time and costs the patient a fair amount of heat, fluid, and blood due to the large abraded surface of lung. The lung is inevitably somewhat battered during the procedure, and a certain amount of third-space fluid loss will occur postoperatively.

Relief of an effusion, a chronic pneumothorax, or a pleural restriction may improve pulmonary function postoperatively. This is in contrast to pulmonary resections, where pulmonary function will always worsen.

In terms of positioning, lung isolation, and postoperative pain, this case is very similar to a pulmonary resection. Read the preceding sections for more pointers.

This procedure is not only incredibly painful postoperatively, as are all thoracotomies, but is also very stimulating throughout. The pleurectomy patient needs a working epidural more than most.

Finally, you may need to work with the surgeon during some pleural strippings, alternately inflating and deflating the operative lung to allow a good view of where the lung stops and the pleura begins.

Mediastinal Mass Excision

Description: Through a median sternotomy the surgeon opens the anterior mediastinum and removes the mass in question, taking the time to dissect it free from any nerves, arteries, veins, airways, or cardiac tissue that it happens to incorporate.

Position:	Supine
Estimated time:	3 hours
Estimated blood loss:	500 ml; type and cross-match 2 units
Need for muscle relaxation:	Helpful*
Indicated monitors:	Standard, A-line, Foley
Postoperative analgesia:	III
Acceptable techniques:	GETA, combined

Comments: Mediastinal tumors can be benign or malignant and can span a wide range of patient ages and conditions. Most tumors are small and easily removed, but every so often one comes along that will test you severely.

A disaster can occur in any mediastinal case if the surgeon is not careful with the bone saw. The innominate vein, innominate artery, and right atrium are all potentially in the line of fire. Bleeding from any of these sources will change the surgical plan dramatically.

Large mediastinal tumors can compress the airways or great vessels, making the patient extremely unstable when anesthetized. In the worst case the patient must be kept sitting and spontaneously ventilating until the pressure is relieved.

Scraping a large tumor off the pericardium can cause enough inflammation to send the patient into atrial fibrillation, which may take weeks to resolve.

A double-lumen tube is not needed, since the surgeon is not typically planning to get involved with the lung. Pay close attention to what's going on, though, and make sure a chest tube is left behind if either pleural space is entered.

*Thymoma is the most commonly resected mediastinal mass. Many of these patients will have myasthenia gravis and will be having the surgery in the hopes of making it better. Read up on this in a good source (like the thoracic surgery chapter in the text by Barash) and remember this simple clinical principle: Use a short-acting nondepolarizing relaxant in small doses, titrated to a specific nerve stimulator response.

Antireflux Surgery (Belsey Mark IV)

Description: Through a low left-sided thoracotomy the surgeon splits the diaphragm, dissects free the lower esophagus and stomach, and then puts things back where they belong: the stomach on one side of the diaphragm and most of the esophagus on the other. The diaphragmatic hiatus is tightened during closure to make sure everything stays put.

Position:	Right lateral decubitus, flexed, leaning slightly back
Estimated time:	3 hours
Estimated blood loss:	700 ml; type and cross-match 4 units
Need for muscle relaxation:	Required
Indicated monitors:	Standard, A-line, Foley
Postoperative analgesia:	IV
Acceptable techniques:	GETA, combined

Comments: This is the one thoracic approach to hiatal hernia repair and is supposedly better for certain kinds of reflux. It is certainly more painful and causes more impairment of ventilation postoperatively than the transabdominal approach. This operation may become increasingly rare now that the equipment exists for doing Nissen fundoplications through a laparoscope.

The patients are all aspiration risks by definition. Prophylaxis and a rapid-sequence intubation are recommended.

The surgeon may ask that you pass a bougie dilator down the esophagus, giving him or her a stent for tightening around.

The large incision necessary for this operation will leak heat and fluid at an amazing rate. You will need to work hard to keep the patient warm and well hydrated. Consider using an active airway heater, a warming blanket, and a fluid warmer.

Single-lung ventilation is required to protect the left lung from battering during the dissection and repair. A double-lumen tube on either side or a tube with a built-in blocker can be used to achieve this.

In terms of position, incision, and postoperative pain, this operation is similar to a thoracotomy for pulmonary resection; read that section for more information.

Transthoracic Esophageal Resection

Description: The esophagus is accessed in one of several ways: through the left chest for low-lying lesions; through the abdomen and right chest (two incisions) for mid-esophageal lesions; and through the right chest, abdomen, and neck (three incisions) for mid- to high esophageal lesions. In any case the proximal stomach and entire esophagus are dissected free, the lesion is removed with an appropriate margin, and the remaining esophagus is connected to the remaining portion of stomach, which will be dissected out with enough of an omentum so that it can be pulled up into the chest.

Position:	Semi-lateral
Estimated time:	8 hours
Estimated blood loss:	2,000 ml; type and cross-match 6 units
Need for muscle relaxation:	Required
Indicated monitors:	Standard, Foley, A-line, CVP/PA lines
Postoperative analgesia:	IV
Acceptable techniques:	GETA, combined

Comments: Make sure you understand what approach the surgeons are contemplating since it will profoundly affect your anesthetic. Then take a good, long look at the patient. Most victims of esophageal carcinoma will be in pretty bad shape. They may be significantly malnourished and may have depleted serum albumin and depleted reserves of clotting factors. Plan to read the section on cancer in Chapter 1. Also read the section on pulmonary resection in this chapter; it outlines many of the routine concerns for this sort of surgery.

Lung isolation is required for any approach going through the left or right chest. A so-called "transhiatal esophagectomy," done for early cancers or benign disease of the esophagus, uses just a neck incision and an abdominal incision with blunt dissection between the two. In addition to a temporary impairment of cardiac filling and blood pressure when the surgeon is bluntly dissecting up behind the heart, there can also be arterial bleeders created that are not easily detected. Have a low threshold for opening the chest if things don't look right.

Fluid shifts and heat loss are impressive during esophageal surgery. Be prepared with plenty of IV access, an active airway heater, and a good blood warmer.

Because of the lengthy nature of the case, the high fluid requirements of the patient, and the risk of postoperative aspiration caused by a high anastomosis, you should plan to leave the patient intubated. Give the swelling around the anastomosis a chance to resolve, let the patient mobilize all of the third-space losses, and then extubate when everything is perfect.

Tracheal Resection

Description: After a rigid bronchoscopy to establish landmarks, the neck is opened transversely and the trachea is dissected free of any surrounding tissue. The diseased segment is removed and the remaining portions are reconnected. The neck is then closed. Sounds easy, doesn't it?

Position:	Supine, head back, shoulders on a roll, arms tucked
Estimated time:	3 hours
Estimated blood loss:	200 ml; type and cross-match 2 units
Need for muscle relaxation:	Not necessary
Indicated monitors:	Standard, A-line, Foley
Postoperative analgesia:	II
Acceptable techniques:	GETA

Comments: This operation is usually done for benign tracheal stenosis and, less commonly, for a carcinoid or similar tumor. The patient may have significant narrowing of the airway preoperatively that can make the initial induction of anesthesia quite dicey. An inhalational induction using a volatile anesthetic allows the patient to continue breathing spontaneously even at a very deep plane of anesthesia and makes the rigid bronchoscopy easy. Jet ventilation is another option. Just remember not to burn any bridges: Test the patient's mask airway carefully before taking it over, and let the surgeon make the initial reconnaissance of the airway using the rigid bronchoscope.

Throughout the operation there will be numerous interruptions of ventilation as the surgeon works around the trachea and your tube. Be sympathetic to the surgeon's needs, but don't be afraid to speak up if the patient is desaturating.

Once the trachea is divided the surgeon will place a flexible, armored endotracheal tube in the lower end and you will be able to hook up to that on the surgical field with a sterile anesthesia circuit prepared in advance. The surgeon will do the resection and the back wall of the anastomosis, and will then ask you to pass an endotracheal tube from above. The surgeon will guide it across the repair and into the distal trachea (having removed the previous tube) and will then close the anterior trachea over your tube. Flexing the head sharply forward will make this easier to do. The rest of the neck is closed, and the patient is left with a large retention stitch in place, holding the chin down to the chest and allowing the trachea to heal without tension.

Despite this awkward position, the surgeon would usually prefer that the patient be extubated at the end of the procedure, since this removes the tube from the vicinity of the suture line. Fluid shifts are usually small during this case, and postoperative pain is minimal so wake-ups are not too hard to accomplish. Just make sure the patient is wide awake and well suctioned out before extubating, though; reintubation will require a flexible bronchoscope.

Cardiac Surgery

Paul F. Lennon

This is the most complicated chapter in the book and the hardest one to write. It can't include everything; it can't even cover all the essentials. Read on, and also read elsewhere.

The challenge of caring for a cardiac surgical patient is that an error—surgical or anesthetic—can be very serious, even fatal. In your favor, however, is that you usually are loaded for bear when you enter the OR. There are many resources to draw on and if all else fails, cardiopulmonary bypass (CPB) is an option. A 2-month rotation in cardiac anesthesia will probably give you the most intense 2 months of your residency. At the end of the rotation, you will be a much better anesthesiologist.

Cardiac patients are as sick as any you might care to meet. Although they have the theoretical advantage of having their heart "fixed" during surgery, this improvement is countered by the immediate insults heaped on their heart by an ischemic arrest and various surgical trespasses. As a result one set of problems is usually traded for another set of problems.

Cardiac operations are highly technical, ritualistic experiences that on a good day feel like a fine ballet. On a bad day—and you'll have some—they'll feel like you're playing tackle football against the Chicago Bears. Alone. Without pads. And the cardiac surgeon will not be out to make your life any better. These detail-oriented perfectionists make the average Marine drill instructor look like a 6-year-old on the first day of school, and they'll be happy to make you feel that way too if you screw up their routine. Try to be sympathetic; they can get into deep trouble fast. Keep a low profile when starting out, and pay attention to what your staff anesthesiologist tells you to do.

Any technique of general anesthesia can be used for these operations; no particular technique has been shown to result in a better outcome. A common and relatively simple approach for cases involving CPB is a high-dose narcotic technique for induction and maintenance.

This technique has the advantages of blunting, or even abolishing, most hemodynamic responses to stimuli while at the same time minimizing anesthetic-induced myocardial depression.

The heart is accessed via a median sternotomy. The sternum is first split with a specially designed saw that can, even with the lungs deflated and the chest immobile, find its way into the innominate vein or right ventricle. The sternum is then pried open with a specialized spreader. This provides good access to the anterior mediastinum and results in—believe it or not—less postoperative pain than a lateral thoracotomy.

CPB is required for most cardiac surgical operations. This allows a relatively motionless heart and therefore does not require the surgeon to chase a moving target. In addition, even if the surgeon could work on a beating heart, the heart doesn't work too well when turned upside down, compressed, or sliced open. CPB also allows, via a heat exchanger, the body to be cooled (and warmed). During CPB, the patient (and heart) is usually cooled; this lowers the metabolic rate and oxygen demand. Prior to separating from CPB the patient is warmed and normothermia restored.

As stated before, to operate on the heart, it needs to be still. Myocardial blood flow is first interrupted with an aortic cross-clamp. Cardioplegia, a cold electrolyte solution high in potassium, is then infused into the coronary circulation. This induces asystole and cools the myocardium, both of which lower oxygen demand. When blood is added to cardioplegia it also increases oxygen supply. Eventually, for function to be restored the heart must be rewarmed and the cardioplegia washed out. This happens with removal of the aortic cross-clamp.

With these basic facts in mind, continue on. However, remember that what makes an anesthesiologist a good cardiac anesthesiologist is attention to basics. One must be both compulsive and flexible. In addition, vigilance cannot be overemphasized. The operative course of these patients, no matter how healthy they appear, can become very dynamic. These patients are notorious for unexpectedly heading south, especially while you are looking the other way.

Cardiopulmonary Bypass

Most cardiac surgical procedures involve the use of CPB. There are some cardiac surgical procedures that do not require CPB; those are procedures that do not require a motionless heart and can be performed without compromising cardiac function (e.g., take-back for bleeding). In general, anesthesia for cardiac surgery can usually be divided into getting a patient to CPB (i.e., lines, induction, surgical dissection, cannulation) and separating the patient from CPB.

Technically the process of CPB is simple: Blood is allowed to drain (via gravity) from the right atrium into a reservoir in the CPB apparatus. From this reservoir a pump moves it through an oxygenator where oxygen is added, carbon dioxide is removed, and blood is warmed (or cooled). This blood is then returned to the patient via a large arterial line usually placed in the proximal ascending aorta. While using a CPB circuit, a surgeon can manipulate and operate on the heart and lungs without limitation. However, by the time the surgeon is finished the heart and lungs must work well enough for CPB to be discontinued.

Although CPB solves many problems by temporarily substituting for the heart and lungs, it creates problems of its own. For example, aortic cannulation may cause atherosclerotic emboli; those can wind up producing ischemic phenomena anywhere in the body, including the brain. Cannulation can also result in aortic dissection. In general, CPB results in injury to every organ system, including the kidneys, lungs, and brain. The severity of the injury is roughly proportional to the length of time during which CPB is employed. CPB requires anticoagulation; this is provided by heparin and—after separation from CPB—is "reversed" with protamine. However, a coagulopathy usually remains as a result of diminished platelet function and, less important, diminished platelet number.

One good way to think about CPB is with the three checklist approach:

PRE-CARDIOPULMONARY BYPASS

1. **Patients must be adequately anticoagulated prior to CPB or they will die.** An activated clotting time (ACT) of greater than 300 seconds is required, and more than 400 seconds is preferred. A heparin dose of 300 U/kg is often sufficient (more if the patient has been on IV heparin). If there is not enough time to wait for the result of the ACT, better to estimate on the high side and give a larger dose of heparin (400 U/kg).

2. Carefully achieve normotension to mild hypotension (systolic blood pressure 85–100 mm Hg) during aortic cannulation, even if this may be lower than optimal for the patient's cardiac disease.

3. Ensure complete muscle relaxation with muscle relaxants.

4. Ensure adequate analgesia and amnesia. Note that hypothermia to less than 31°C is an excellent amnestic.

5. Empty the Foley catheter.

6. Withdraw the PA catheter 5 cm.

7. Check the pupils (for baseline).

ON CARDIOPULMONARY BYPASS

1. Turn off all inhalational anesthetics.

2. Stop ventilating the patient once CPB is flowing.

3. Turn off all drug infusions and IV fluid infusions. Any IV drugs or fluids needed during this interval can be administered by the perfusionist into the CPB apparatus.

4. Communicate with the perfusionist. He or she will attempt to maintain total CPB flow and arterial blood pressure within predetermined ranges. Occasionally, a vasodilator or vasoconstrictor may be needed. Anesthetics and vasoactive drugs can be used through the CPB machine, including volatile anesthetics given by a vaporizer.

5. Check the face. Plethora may indicate an obstruction to superior vena cava (SVC) outflow.

6. Examine the eyes for pupil symmetry and size. New asymmetry may indicate a misdirected inflow cannula that is perfusing one carotid more than the other carotid.

7. **Maintain adequate anticoagulation or the**

patient will die. Protocols vary at different institutions. Some follow the ACT. Others dose heparin on a fixed schedule. Regardless of the method used to determine the need for heparin, more will probably have to be given before you finish.

8. Check an arterial blood gas (ABG) and hematocrit every 30 minutes. A hematocrit as low as 15–18 may be tolerable during CPB and hypothermia.

9. Monitor urine output.

SEPARATION FROM CARDIOPULMONARY BYPASS

1. Confirm that adequate warming (>35°C rectal) has occurred.

2. Start ventilating the patient. Initially hand ventilate to reverse any gross atelectasis and to ensure that, if an internal mammary artery was used for grafting, it has enough "slack" (i.e., is not pulled off the heart by an inflated lung).

3. Confirm acceptable laboratory values including hematocrit, blood gas, calcium, and potassium. Depending on the clinical situation, a hematocrit of 18–20 may be sufficient.

4. Confirm that a functional temporary pacemaker is available. Consider pacing if the heart rate is less than 80.

5. Correct arrhythmias. Note that even patients with chronic atrial fibrillation can sometimes be cardioverted.

6. Consider the administration of inotropes and/or vasopressors. This decision is based on many factors, including the preoperative condition of the heart, the length of the ischemic (aortic cross-clamp) time interval, the adequacy of myocardial protection, the adequacy of the surgical intervention, and, immediately prior to separation from CPB, the appearance of the heart and state of systemic arterial tone. The administration and selection of hemodynamic agents is often based on discussion with the surgeons. Their input can be both instructive and politically wise.

7. Gradually discontinue CPB. The surgeon initiates this by clamping the venous cannula, preventing

drainage of venous blood into the CPB apparatus. The perfusionist decreases and then discontinues blood flow into the aortic cannula from the CPB apparatus. Blood is added via the aortic cannula until an adequate volume status is achieved.

8. Assess the patient's hemodynamic status. Adequate myocardial function can be assessed by visual inspection of the heart and measuring a cardiac output (via thermodilution). If the patient is hypotensive with a normal to high cardiac index, a vasopressor may be necessary. If the patient is hypotensive with a low cardiac index, an inotrope may be necessary (after again confirming adequate volume status).

9. Just to confuse things, immediately after separation from CPB, arterial pressure measured from a radial arterial line is frequently substantially lower than aortic pressure. Although this often corrects after 30 minutes, adequate measurement of arterial pressure in this interval can be challenging. Alternatives include a femoral or brachial arterial line, a temporary aortic line, and transducing the aortic cannula.

10. If hemodynamics are acceptable and after discussion with the surgeon, administer protamine to reverse the effect of heparin. One milligram of protamine reverses 100 U active heparin. The dose of heparin can be estimated (taking the half-life of heparin into account); some centers use devices like the Hepcon to calculate the dose. In any case, serial ACTs are followed.

11. Administer protamine slowly (i.e., over at least 10 minutes), preferably after dilution. Hemodynamic sequelae of protamine administration can include anaphylaxis, systemic hypotension, and pulmonary arterial vasoconstriction. Be ready to halt its administration and support the circulation. Have heparin readily available.

12. An ongoing intravascular volume requirement is common. Request the perfusionist to add volume via the aortic cannula (if still in place). After the cannula is removed, make use of your large-bore IV access.

13. The surgeon will remove the venous cannula, followed by the aortic cannula.

14. After protamine administration is complete, check an ACT and observe the surgical field for evidence of

blood clot. Evaluation and treatment of ongoing bleeding is beyond the scope of this book but often includes continued surgical exploration, additional protamine, laboratory testing, and blood product administration (especially platelets).

15. Prepare yourself for transport to the ICU with a fistful of emergency drugs, a pacemaker, a bag and mask ventilation system, oxygen, and a good monitor.

Coronary Artery Bypass Surgery (CABG)

Description: After opening the chest, dissecting out a saphenous vein(s) and/or an internal mammary artery, establishing CPB, and cooling the patient, the surgeon places vascular grafts to the distal coronary arteries. These grafts result in an increase in blood flow distal to the "bypassed" coronary artery stenosis. If a vein graft is used, the proximal ends of the grafts are anastomosed (end-to-side) to the ascending aorta. If the internal mammary artery is used, its proximal end remains attached where it belongs. Once all the grafts are attached, CPB is discontinued, the chest is closed, and the patient is taken to the ICU.

Position:	Supine, arms out or at side
Estimated time:	4 hours
Estimated blood loss:	2,000 ml; type and cross-match 3 units
Need for muscle relaxation:	Yes
Indicated monitors:	Standard, Foley, A-line, PA line, frequent labs
Postoperative analgesia:	III
Acceptable techniques:	GETA

Comments: This operation is performed more than any other operation in the United States. It may be relatively routine in a patient with discrete proximal coronary artery stenoses and well-preserved myocardial function. On the other hand, in a patient with failing myocardium and distal coronary artery occlusions, this surgery may be extremely challenging.

Place at least one peripheral large-bore (e.g., 16-gauge or 14-gauge) IV catheter and a radial arterial line. Central access is required for the administration of vasoactive drugs; central pressure monitoring is also extremely helpful. Therefore, a PA catheter is usually placed. The central line is also needed for the administration of vasoactive drug infusions. Confirm the presence of functional drug infusion devices and be familiar with their organization and operation.

During induction of anesthesia and prior to CPB, the goal is to reduce or prevent coronary ischemia. Avoid increases in myocardial oxygen demand by maintaining a heart rate less than 70–80 per minute. Avoid a decrease in myocardial oxygen supply by maintaining normotension (i.e., mean arterial pressure [MAP] >65 mm Hg). Episodes of myocardial ischemia can be treated by optimizing hemodynamics and, if arterial blood pressure permits, by IV administration of nitroglycerin. Since MAP tends to go down rather than up with induction, have a vasopressor readily available.

Dissection ("taking down") the internal mammary artery is done before establishing bypass and typically adds 30 minutes to the procedure. Smaller ventilator tidal volumes (with an increased rate) or even manual ventilation may be helpful during this interval to optimize surgical conditions. Surgical stimulation is minimal during this period, and the patient may need hemodynamic support or less anesthesia.

Although the operation is potentially very helpful and may be life-saving, the heart rarely works as well immediately following CABG as it did prior to CABG. Inotropic support may be necessary, especially if myocardial function was marginal prior to surgery.

Mitral Valve Replacement (MVR)

Description: After induction, sternotomy, cannulation, CPB, and cooling, the heart is opened via the left atrium. The diseased mitral valve is excised and a prosthetic valve placed. The heart is then purged of air and closed. The patient is warmed and separated from CPB.

Position:	Supine, arms out or at side
Estimated time:	4 hours
Estimated blood loss:	2,000 ml; type and cross-match 3 units
Need for muscle relaxation:	Required
Indicated monitors:	Standard, Foley, A-line, PA catheter; consider TEE
Postoperative analgesia:	III
Acceptable techniques:	GETA

Comments: Mitral valve replacement is required to correct mitral stenosis and/or insufficiency. The former is usually due to rheumatic heart disease; the latter has many possible causes, including endocarditis and papillary muscle dysfunction.

Preoperatively, be judicious with the use of premedication. These patients tend to be especially sensitive to sedatives. In patients with mitral regurgitation, be especially wary of those with a reduced ejection fraction (EF). Reduction in the EF in the presence of mitral regurgitation suggests marked depression of left ventricular function.

When placing a pulmonary artery catheter, be careful of obtaining a "wedge" pressure trace. Accompanying pulmonary hypertension places these patients at increased risk of pulmonary artery rupture. In addition, in patients with mitral regurgitation a prominent V-wave may be present. This may make it difficult to recognize the transition from a pulmonary arterial to a wedge pressure trace.

Patients with mitral stenosis will benefit if tachycardia is avoided, adequate preload is maintained, and sinus rhythm is preserved; all these maneuvers encourage increased blood flow across the stenotic valve. Be careful with induction; any vasopressor you administer for hypotension may also exacerbate pre-existing pulmonary hypertension or lead to deleterious increases in heart rate.

Patients with mitral insufficiency will benefit from a normal or slightly elevated heart rate and a normal or slightly decreased systemic vascular resistance; both of these maneuvers reduce the regurgitant volume. An infusion of dopamine at a low rate can produce both of these hemodynamic effects and should be readily available. If the patient is markedly compromised, consider initiating a dopamine infusion prior to induction.

After mitral valve replacement and CPB, a low normal mean arterial blood pressure is usually sufficient. Avoid marked arterial hypertension; it can place undue stress on the new valve, the suture line, the left ventricle, and your residency.

Mitral valve surgery is an ideal case for using transesophageal echocardiography (TEE); it provides a superb view of the left atrium and mitral valve. The function of the native valve (prior to CPB) and the new valve (after CPB) can easily be evaluated. In cases of mitral valve repair, a TEE is almost mandatory.

Aortic Valve Replacement (AVR)

Description: After the usual open heart start, the aorta is opened and the diseased valve removed. A new valve is placed, either mechanical or porcine; the heart is closed and purged of air. The patient is warmed and separated from CPB.

Position:	Supine
Estimated time:	4 hours
Estimated blood loss:	2,000 ml; type and cross-match 3 units
Need for muscle relaxation:	Required
Indicated monitors:	Standard, Foley, A-line, PA catheter; consider TEE
Postoperative analgesia:	III
Acceptable techniques:	GETA

Comments: Aortic valve replacement is required to correct aortic stenosis or insufficiency. The former is usually due to rheumatic heart disease, a congenitally bicuspid valve, or senile degeneration. The latter can be due to numerous causes, including rheumatic heart disease and endocarditis.

A patient with aortic stenosis has an obstruction to outflow from the left ventricle. The degree of obstruction is usually expressed as a valve area (calculated from the Gorlin equation using measurements of pressure and flow) and the peak systolic pressure gradient (from left ventricle to aorta). In general, the degree of obstruction increases with a decrease in the valve area or an increase in the gradient. A valve area less than 0.4 cm^2 or a gradient more than 50 mm Hg is considered critical.

A patient with aortic stenosis may present with angina, syncope, or heart failure. The urgency for replacement increases with the appearance, in the above order, of these symptoms. Note that coronary artery disease need not be present for angina to occur. The oxygen demands of the hypertrophied myocardium can outstrip the supply of even an unobstructed coronary arterial system.

Patients with aortic stenosis, more than most, require maintenance of systemic pressure to perfuse the myocardium. Systemic arterial vasodilation and hypotension must be avoided and if they occur, they must be quickly and aggressively treated. A vasopressor such as phenylephrine or norepinephrine should be readily available. These patients especially benefit from a slow and controlled induction. Onset of atrial fibrillation is poorly tolerated and may need to be aggressively treated.

Patients with aortic insufficiency, as with mitral regurgitation, will benefit from a normal or slightly elevated heart rate and a normal or slightly decreased systemic vascular resistance. Also, a dopamine infusion can be very helpful with these patients. A complete and reassuring preoperative visit combined with judicious use of premedication is extremely important. A surge in anxiety (and a surge in blood pressure) may be poorly tolerated when the patient arrives in the OR.

A PA line provides extremely valuable information in patients requiring aortic valve replacement, especially after CPB. In particular, patients with prior aortic stenosis usually have hypertrophied, poorly compliant left ventricles. Ventricular compliance is further decreased immediately after CPB, and as a result these patients often require high filling pressures.

After CPB avoid systemic arterial hypertension. In addition to the aortic cannulation site there is an aortotomy site through which the aortic valve was accessed. Hypertension also places added stress on the new aortic valve. Vigilance is especially important here as blood pressure may be very labile, especially in patients with prior aortic stenosis.

A TEE may be useful in assessing the adequacy of purging air from the heart and left ventricular filling. However, it may be less than ideal for the evaluation of aortic valve function.

Combined Valve Replacement and CABG

Description: The distal vein grafts are usually sewn on first. After the valve is replaced, the heart is closed and purged of air. The aortic cross-clamp is removed, the patient is warmed, the proximal vein grafts are placed, and the patient is separated from CPB.

Position:	Supine, arms either out or at side
Estimated time:	7 hours
Estimated blood loss:	3,000 ml; type and cross-match 4 units
Need for muscle relaxation:	Required
Indicated monitors:	Standard, Foley, A-line, PA catheter; consider TEE
Postoperative analgesia:	III
Acceptable techniques:	GETA

Comments: The patient's coronary disease can be of varying severity. On the one hand, it may not be severe enough by itself to warrant heart surgery and CABG. However, because the patient will be undergoing cardiac surgery for valve replacement a CABG is also done. On the other hand, the patient may be very ill and have severe, multivessel coronary disease and severe valvular disease. In addition, coronary disease that permits normal daily life may, unless corrected, prevent separation from CPB.

These patients benefit from a controlled induction. The hemodynamic goals for the patient's valvular disease may not be the same as those for the patient's coronary disease. It's probably best to focus on the more significant disease and manage accordingly. However, your best bet may be to keep the patient as close as possible to his or her preoperative baseline.

A combined procedure usually means a longer CPB time, longer aortic cross-clamp time, and all the bad things that go along with these: myocardial dysfunction, platelet consumption and dysfunction, and pulmonary injury.

Bleeding is apt to be more pronounced because of the longer CPB time and the multiple surgical sites. Consider placing two large-bore peripheral IVs preoperatively. You should be prepared with additional venous access; blood products should also be readily available.

Re-Do CABG

Description: This is a CABG after the patient has had at least one previous CABG (usually years prior to the current surgery). The major problem with the surgery is that it requires dissection through and operating within a morass of scar tissue; this is tedious and is fraught with hazard. Other than that, the procedure is the same as a CABG (although adequate conduit for the bypass grafts may be harder to find).

Position:	Supine, arms out or at side
Estimated time:	7 hours
Estimated blood loss:	4,000 ml; type and cross-match 6 units
Need for muscle relaxation:	Yes
Indicated monitors:	Standard, Foley, A-line, PA catheter, frequent labs
Postoperative analgesia:	III
Acceptable techniques:	GETA

Comments: Because a CABG is the most commonly performed operation in the United States and because its benefits are time-limited, it is not surprising that the number of "re-do" CABGs is increasing. With advances in surgical and anesthetic skills and improvements in perioperative care, there is also less hesitancy to do these operations. Previously confined mostly to high-volume tertiary care centers, this operation will soon be common in every cardiac surgical practice.

In addition to the usual potential problems with a CABG patient, there are additional problems with a re-do CABG. These patients usually have sicker hearts. Surgical dissection can interrupt or cause emboli in existing grafts and may result in ischemia with impaired myocardial function, conduction disturbances, and arrhythmias. If hemodynamic problems occur, the surgeon may not be able to quickly cannulate and begin CPB. Adequate delivery of cardioplegia may be difficult, resulting in poor myocardial protection. Aortic cross-clamp and CPB times are longer, and after separation from CPB, bleeding tends to be greater due to the increased CPB time and dissection of scar tissue.

Place adequate venous access; usually two large-bore peripheral IVs are sufficient (in addition to central access). Some anesthesiologists prefer to place PA catheters with ventricular pacing capability; you may be able to pace if complete heart block occurs during surgical dissection. Always have blood available (and checked) in the room prior to sternotomy. Be ready to assist the surgeon by manually ventilating the lungs during surgical dissection.

Be especially careful in the management of these patients. If hemodynamic problems occur, the surgeon can't save the day by quickly initiating CPB. Arrhythmias requiring cardioversion or defibrillation prior to dissection of the heart can be problematic. Internal paddles may not be able to be adequately positioned. Confirm prior to prepping that a workable plan exists for (sterile) external cardioversion or defibrillation (e.g., sterile external paddles).

Ascending Aorta or Aortic Arch Surgery

Description: CPB is established and the patient is cooled. The diseased segment of the aorta is excised and, if necessary, replaced with a prosthesis. If surgery involves the aortic arch, deep hypothermic circulatory arrest (DHCA) may be used. After the repair, the patient is warmed and separated from CPB.

Position:	Supine
Estimated time:	6 hours
Estimated blood loss:	4,000 ml; type and cross-match 8 units; consider platelets and fresh-frozen plasma
Need for muscle relaxation:	Required
Indicated monitors:	Standard, Foley, A-line(s), PA catheter; consider TEE
Postoperative analgesia:	IV
Acceptable techniques:	GETA

Comments: Ascending or aortic arch surgery is relatively uncommon and usually is performed for an aneurysm or a dissection. This type of surgery tends to be performed at centers with a high cardiac surgical volume. It also tends to result in a significant rate of morbidity and mortality, particularly if it involves the aortic arch. Repair of aneurysms usually involves replacement of the diseased segment. Repair of a dissection may be limited to excision (and possible replacement) of the segment containing the intimal tear. Thoracic aortic aneurysms can occur from medionecrosis, tertiary syphilis, Kawasaki disease, Marfan syndrome, and atherosclerosis. Thoracic aortic dissections are largely due to hypertension. If the aortic valve annulus is involved, replacement of the aortic valve may also be necessary.

The arterial line should be placed in an artery whose flow does not depend on the segment of the aorta to be clamped and excised. Discuss this with the surgeon beforehand. For ascending aortic surgery, place it in the femoral or left radial artery. For aortic arch surgery, you may only be able to use a femoral site. Note that aortic cannulation for CPB in these cases is usually via the femoral artery. However, for cases restricted to the ascending thoracic aorta, cannulation may be possible immediately distal to the aortic repair.

Induction of anesthesia should be approached as for any cardiac surgical case. Be aware of possible associated aortic insufficiency. Aneurysms and dissections can worsen with severe hypertension; don't let this happen.

These cases tend to have a lot of bleeding. The cause may not be readily apparent but can include a long CPB time, DHCA, and two or more aortic suture lines. Always be prepared with an abundance of IV access, an adequate supply of blood products (including platelets and fresh-frozen plasma), and extra help available to administer it.

If surgery involves interruption of the cerebral blood supply (e.g., aortic arch reconstruction), DHCA may be necessary. The goal in this technique is to lower body temperature and thereby lower the patient's metabolic rate and oxygen demand to the point where blood flow (and oxygen delivery) can be completely stopped. In this technique, the patient is cooled to a very low temperature (15–20°C), the blood is drained into the CPB reservoir, and CPB is stopped. Closed bags of ice can be applied to the head to assist in brain cooling. In an effort to further reduce the incidence of central nervous system (CNS) injury, some centers advocate the administration of various medications (e.g., mannitol, methylpred-nisolone, sodium thiopental) immediately prior to DHCA. During DHCA, blood flow (including cerebral blood flow) may be able to be interrupted for up to 60 minutes without permanent clinical sequelae. Disadvantages to this technique include CNS injury, even with an arrest time of less than 60 minutes, increased CPB time due to prolonged cooling (and warming), and bleeding.

Automatic Internal Cardiac Defibrillator (AICD) Placement

Description: With improvements in technology, this procedure has changed several times in the last few years; it will probably continue to change in the coming years. The basic idea is to place defibrillator electrodes in contact with the myocardium and connect them via leads to a small box (generator) containing the energy source and intelligent circuitry. This box is placed in a subcutaneous pocket usually just caudad to the ribs on the left side.

Position:	Supine/right lateral decubitus
Estimated time:	3 hours
Estimated blood loss:	300 ml; type and cross-match 2 units
Need for muscle relaxation:	Required
Indicated monitors:	Standard, Foley, A-line; consider CVP or PA line
Postoperative analgesia:	II
Acceptable techniques:	GETA, combined

Comments: These devices are implanted in patients with a suspected or proven history of hemodynamically significant arrhythmias, usually ventricular fibrillation (VF) or ventricular tachycardia (VT). The device can sense VF or VT and in response deliver an electrical discharge resulting in defibrillation or synchronized cardioversion, respectively. During surgery to place the AICD, VT or VF is induced, often repeatedly, to test the device's effectiveness. In the past both defibrillator electrodes were wire pads and were surgically placed on the epicardium via a left lateral thoracotomy. Recent improvements in technique and hardware may allow subcutaneous placement of one electrode or percutaneous endocardial placement of one or both electrodes.

Other than a history of arrhythmias, the patient's heart may be relatively normal. However, refractory ventricular arrhythmias are common in patients with impaired ventricular function. Although the patient may have a significant degree of coronary artery disease, any potential myocardial ischemic disease is usually corrected by a prior or concomitant CABG.

Essentially the placement and testing of the device involves repeated (as many as 30!) intentional cardiac arrests (electrically induced), each followed by a resuscitation. Resuscitation is usually accomplished solely by cardioversion or defibrillation by the AICD.

An arterial line is invaluable during the procedure due to the frequent intentionally induced episodes of VT or VF. For the same reason, central venous access can also be invaluable, especially for drug administration. A PA line may be needed in compromised patients (e.g., moderate to severe congestive heart failure [CHF]).

If a thoracotomy is planned, general anesthesia is used. Preoperative placement of a thoracic epidural catheter will help with postop analgesia and may also be used intraop. Most patients can be awakened and extubated either at the end of the procedure or shortly after arrival in the ICU. After placement, the device is often turned off while the surgery is completed. Make sure you always know the status of the device!

Always be prepared for the AICD not to function effectively. Place external defibrillation pads before beginning the procedure. Confirm that a functional defibrillator is present and that you are familiar with its use. Also, have readily available any drugs (e.g., epinephrine, lidocaine, procainamide) that you might need. You will have a hard time explaining later why you were unprepared for a cardiac arrest!

Expect additional personnel (e.g., cardiologist, technician, nurse, company representative) in the room.

Cardiac Take-Back for Bleeding

Description: This procedure is pretty much self-explanatory. The surgeon calls and tells you that the open heart you did earlier in the day never stopped bleeding and needs to be explored. Back in the OR, the surgeon will reopen the sternum, evacuate any clot, and look around for the bleeding point(s). If it involves the heart, CPB may be needed. Fortunately, this is uncommon. Many times, the bleeding site(s) can be identified and fixed with electrocautery and suture. Occasionally, the cause for ongoing bleeding cannot be identified with certainty.

Position:	Supine
Estimated time:	Indeterminate
Estimated blood loss:	1,000 ml; type and cross-match 6 units; consider fresh-frozen plasma and platelets
Need for muscle relaxation:	Required
Indicated monitors:	Standard, Foley, A-line, PA catheter
Postoperative analgesia:	III
Acceptable techniques:	GETA

Comments: No one likes this operation. It usually occurs late in the day or at night. People are tired and it is difficult to transport a patient who may be hemodynamically tenuous with multiple lines, infusions, and tubes. Attempts are usually first made in the ICU to aggressively correct any proven (or suspected) coagulopathy prior to returning to the OR. However, if bleeding is suspected of causing hemodynamic compromise (e.g., tamponade), a return to the OR should not be delayed. If hemodynamic collapse is severe, a trip to the OR may have to wait until after the chest is opened in the ICU by the cardiothoracic surgeon.

Bleeding after cardiac surgery and CPB can have numerous causes. There is surgical bleeding (e.g., a hole in a blood vessel), and there is nonsurgical bleeding (i.e., coagulopathy). Reasons for a coagulopathy can include the preoperative use of drugs (e.g., aspirin, crystalline warfarin sodium [Coumadin]), platelet dysfunction, residual heparin, residual hypothermia, and consumption of coagulation factors. Institutions may have criteria for a return to the OR based on the amount of chest and mediastinal drainage. Rigid adherence to these criteria is not the norm, but blood loss of more than 200 ml per hour usually means a return to the OR for a look around.

On arrival at the patient's bedside, quickly learn the current hemodynamics, lines, and drug infusions. You must know this information! Write it on your scrubs if necessary. Speak with the patient's nurse for the most up-to-date information. Confirm that the blood bank has products available; request blood products if needed. Before traveling to the OR, make sure that you have transport monitoring, oxygen, and a means of delivering positive pressure ventilation. Also, have a source of intravascular volume (preferably blood) and a good IV line. And finally, do not rely solely on the patient's drug infusions. Bring vasoactive drugs, in syringe form, with you.

This is a case where flexibility is needed. There may or may not be an urgency to the situation. Use available time to learn more about the patient and prepare for transport. If the situation is urgent, you may have to act quickly. Again, at least know the patient's hemodynamics, lines, and drug infusions. Most of the battle with a cardiac take-back is getting the patient from the ICU to the OR while maintaining a stable hemodynamic state and without losing any lines.

Seek more IV access if you need it. Fortunately, the lines placed for the original case are usually sufficient. A decrease in the pressor or inotrope requirement usually occurs after the sternum is opened as clot or blood is evacuated. Aggressive blood component replacement therapy may be needed and should, as best as can be done, be guided by laboratory studies.

Percutaneous Transluminal Coronary Angioplasty (PTCA)/Atherectomy

Description: A cardiologist threads a special catheter, via the patient's groin, across a stenotic or occluded segment of a coronary artery. This catheter may have a balloon that is then inflated and results in dilation of the diseased segment (PTCA). Alternatively, the catheter may be able to excise, via a rotary cutting device, the intraluminal obstruction (atherectomy). This procedure takes place in the cardiac catheterization lab. You are usually called when the procedure makes things worse rather than better.

Position:	Supine
Estimated time:	60 minutes
Estimated blood loss:	Minimal
Need for muscle relaxation:	None
Indicated monitors:	Standard
Postoperative analgesia:	II
Acceptable techniques:	Local

Comments: These procedures, although they take place in a catheter lab, are only performed at hospitals where cardiac surgery can be performed. There is a small risk (2–5%) that the patient will need an urgent CABG as a result of the procedure. The most common reason for a CABG in this situation is that the procedure actually worsens the coronary artery obstruction.

The policy for surgical "coverage" is not uniform. One institution may have a cardiac surgical OR open and ready with a team available. Another institution may not set aside any OR and treat the PTCA-gone-bad like any other surgical emergency. Institutions with a large number of cardiac surgical ORs and cardiac surgeons can have the most flexibility. However, even in those institutions, high-risk procedures in selected patients may warrant setting aside an open OR. Likewise, the policy for preoperative assessment is not uniform. Since only a small number of these patients will require an urgent visit to the OR, it seems unreasonable for an anesthesiologist to interview and assess every patient prior to the procedure. However, high-risk patients may benefit from such an interview and assessment.

The cardiologist has a number of tools to use if the procedure results in coronary occlusion. Repeated balloon inflations may not be of any help. However, a small catheter may be able to be threaded across the lesion and allow, via its distal tip, blood flow to the jeopardized myocardium. An intra-aortic balloon pump (IABP) can also be placed. This will improve cardiac output and decrease myocardial oxygen supply. Of course, vasoactive drugs (e.g., nitroglycerin, dopamine) can be added.

This is another instance where flexibility is needed. The patient may be close to death with CPR imminent or in progress. On the other hand, the patient may be stable on an IABP and simply need a CABG within the next few hours. Learn as much as you can about the patient as quickly as you can. Triage your assessment. Initially concentrate on hemodynamic status, medications, and lines. The patient will have femoral arterial and venous lines. Do not, do not, do not forget, overlook, or ignore these lines. They may be life-saving.

The OR should be prepared for a CABG. Transport to the OR with supplemental oxygen while monitoring the ECG and femoral arterial blood pressure. Again, familiarize yourself with all lines and rates of drug infusions. Have emergency drugs (e.g., epinephrine, lidocaine) and equipment (e.g., defibrillator, laryngoscope) available. Remember that the patient may be fully awake and very frightened. While obtaining a brief, pertinent medical history, attempt to reassure and explain.

After arrival in the OR, use judgment in proceeding. The femoral arterial line should be transduced and can function as your arterial line. The femoral venous line can be used to administer volume, vasoactive drugs, and heparin. Depending on the urgency of the situation, a peripheral large-bore IV can be placed. A central line can be placed before or after induction. One method is to induce anesthesia and, if the patient is stable, quickly place a central line. If the patient continues to remain stable, continue and place a PA catheter. Always remember that although multiple lines are helpful, only one IV is needed to induce anesthesia, administer heparin, and initiate CPB.

There are usually other anesthesiologists available for assistance. Learn to assign them specific tasks (e.g., obtain peripheral IV access, set up drug infusions).

The patient is almost surely anticoagulated, although not enough for CPB. Remember this when obtaining vascular access and instrumenting the airway.

Pediatric Cardiac Catheterization

Description: The arterial and venous systems are usually cannulated from the groin, and contrast injections are used to define the anatomy of the heart and central vessels.

Position:	Supine
Estimated time:	60 minutes
Estimated blood loss:	100 ml; type and screen
Need for muscle relaxation:	Helpful
Indicated monitors:	Standard
Postoperative analgesia:	II
Acceptable techniques:	MAC, GETA

Comments: Pediatric cardiac catheterization is more likely to occur at institutions that have a pediatric cardiac surgical practice. The pediatric cardiologists are usually adept at sedating and performing these procedures on children. The presence and care of an anesthesiologist is usually requested when the child is particularly difficult to adequately sedate or an interventional procedure (e.g., valvuloplasty) is planned.

Children have cardiac catheterizations to investigate (and sometimes correct) congenital cardiac lesions. Explanations of these lesions and their management is well beyond the scope of this book. These patients are best cared for by an anesthesiologist with an interest in pediatric and/or cardiac anesthesia. However, there are a few general suggestions in dealing with these patients.

Understand the patient's known or suspected cardiac lesion. Read as required and consult liberally. Discuss the patient and the plan for the catheterization with the cardiologist and your staff anesthesiologist.

Remember that general anesthesia may be required to keep the patient still or to ensure adequate ventilation and oxygenation. However, the cardiologist's measurements of vascular pressures and saturations will be altered by GETA and may yield less information. Also, general anesthesia in children with congenital heart disease has considerations specific to their type of disease. Again, learn as much as possible beforehand. Test yourself in preparation by playing out different scenarios in your mind and how you would react to each of them.

Ketamine is preferred in many institutions for sedation. Increased oral secretions can be diminished with prior administration of an antisialagogue (e.g., glycopyrrolate). Note that with ketamine, sedation with airway obstruction or myocardial depression can still occur.

Especially in the case of an interventional procedure, there are specific moments when the child must be still. Anticipate these moments (ask the cardiologist if necessary) and plan your sedation accordingly.

Blood loss can be significant when accounting for the patient's body weight (and blood volume). Attempt to visually monitor blood loss at the site of the catheter insertion. Remember that obtaining a blood sample for a hematocrit and type and screen can be done relatively easily during the catheterization.

Atrial Septal Defect Repair (ASD)

Description: The chest is opened and the superior vena cava (SVC) and inferior vena cava (IVC) (rather than the right atrium) are cannulated. CPB is begun, the aorta is cross-clamped, and cardioplegia is administered. The right atrium is opened and the defect is closed either primarily or with pericardial or synthetic graft. The atrium is closed and the heart is purged of air. The patient is warmed and separated from CPB.

Position:	Supine
Estimated time:	3 hours
Estimated blood loss:	2,000 ml; type and cross-match 3 units
Need for muscle relaxation:	Required
Indicated monitors:	Standard, Foley, A-line, central line; consider TEE
Postoperative analgesia:	III
Acceptable techniques:	GETA

Comments: In general, patients undergoing ASD repairs are healthy. These patients usually have come to medical attention because of an abnormal physical exam (murmur), decreased exercise tolerance (pulmonary congestion), or unexplained stroke (paradoxical embolus). They also tend to be younger than the usual adult cardiac surgical patient.

Normally, the pressure in the right atrium is lower than that in the left atrium. As a result, these patients have a left-to-right shunt whose severity depends on the actual size of the ASD and the respective atrial pressures. In an older patient with a long history of an ASD, this chronic elevation in pulmonary blood flow may have resulted in pulmonary hypertension and reversal to a right-to-left shunt; these patients do not usually come to the OR.

A central line (without a PA line) is placed preoperatively. A PA line is usually avoided because (1) it would be present in the surgical field and (2) these patients usually do not require it for intraoperative or postoperative management. Do not allow any air to enter the IV lines. Any intravenous air may cross from the right atrium to left atrium and result in an arterial air embolus!

Theoretically, any maneuver that decreases pulmonary vascular resistance (e.g., hypocarbia, increase in inspired oxygen) or increased systemic vascular resistance (e.g., vasopressors) may worsen the degree of the underlying left-to-right shunt. However, these patients are usually well compensated at rest. Therefore, induction of anesthesia and management prior to CPB can be managed similar to other patients.

These patients usually separate from CPB without difficulty except in the uncommon case of a prolonged cross-clamp interval or inadequate cardioplegia administration. If myocardial function is poor, suspect coronary artery air emboli or an inadequate repair.

Compared with other patients undergoing cardiac surgery and CPB, these patients tend to be healthier and younger. They also tend to require shorter aortic cross-clamp and CPB times. Therefore, a patient may be able to be awakened and extubated at the end of the case in the OR or shortly after arrival in the ICU. However, be careful. Make sure that the patient is warm, not bleeding, hemodynamically stable, fully awake, and strong.

Descending Thoracic Aortic Surgery

Description: The chest is opened via a left lateral thoracotomy and the descending thoracic aorta is dissected and clamped above and below the involved segment. The clamped aorta is opened, a synthetic graft is sewn in place, and the old aorta is closed over the graft. The clamps are removed, bleeding is controlled, and the chest is closed.

Position:	Right lateral decubitus
Estimated time:	4–6 hours
Estimated blood loss:	2,000 ml; type and cross-match 8 units; consider fresh-frozen plasma and platelets; use autotransfusion device
Need for muscle relaxation:	Required
Indicated monitors:	Standard, Foley, A-line, PA catheter
Postoperative analgesia:	IV
Acceptable techniques:	GETA, epidural for postoperative analgesia

Comments: This surgery may be required for repair of either an aortic dissection or aneurysm. In the descending thoracic aorta, dissections are usually due to pre-existing hypertension, and aneurysms are usually due to atherosclerosis or trauma.

Be prepared for blood loss with generous venous access (at least two large-bore peripheral IVs), blood in the room, and clotting factors readily available. Choose a PA line for your central line for two reasons: (1) the proximal aortic clamp can lead to very impressive hemodynamic changes and (2) partial CPB may be used. Place the arterial line in the right arm (the proximal aortic clamp may involve the left subclavian).

Before placing (and using) an epidural catheter, discuss it beforehand with the surgeon. Remember that (1) full anticoagulation may be necessary intraoperatively, (2) neurologic problems (e.g., paraplegia) occur with this type of surgery, and (3) a postoperative neurologic exam is eagerly awaited by all involved.

Aortic aneurysms and dissections can only get worse with hypertension, increased myocardial contractility, and increased heart rate. Aggressively treat (or better yet, avoid) these hemodynamic boogeymen. A beta blocker may be optimal.

The descending aorta is approached via a left lateral thoracotomy. One-lung ventilation is of immense benefit to the surgeon. A double-lumen endotracheal tube may be best, maybe even a right-sided tube. However, because aortic pathology often distorts tracheobronchial anatomy, placement may be difficult. Regardless of your plan, have options readily available.

With placement of the aortic clamps, impressive hypertension occurs above the proximal clamp (e.g., aortic arch, ascending aorta, carotid arteries), hypotension below the distal clamp (e.g., renal arteries), and no blood pressure between the clamps. Severe hypertension above the clamp can lead to myocardial ischemia; treat it aggressively with vasodilators (e.g., nitroprusside). Severe hypotension below the distal clamp can lead to organ failure (e.g., kidneys). No blood pressure between the clamps (and no blood flow to the intercostal arteries) can lead to spinal cord ischemia and paraplegia.

One surgical technique is to clamp, sew, and move quickly. This can be expanded to include perfusion of the aorta below the distal clamp. A shunt from the proximal aorta to the distal aorta can be placed. Alternatively, a shunt can be placed from the left atrium to the distal aorta (with a pump in between). Another technique is partial CPB via femoral arterial and venous cannulae. Techniques involving a shunt or partial CPB can be very effective in both treating hypertension above the proximal clamp by "unloading" that circulation and also preventing ischemia of organs below the distal clamp.

To prevent or minimize renal failure, give mannitol before the aorta is clamped, especially if a shunt isn't used. Techniques to prevent paraplegia are controversial. Surgical reimplantation of one or more intercostal arteries into the graft may be most beneficial. Other techniques are controversial. These include allowing a lower body temperature (32–34°C), which may permit a longer clamp time (and ischemic interval), and preoperative placement of a lumbar spinal catheter with drainage of CSF during aortic clamping.

When the distal clamp is removed, hypotension is common. (It may be less likely if a shunt is used and is a non-issue if partial CPB is used.) Anticipate this surgical maneuver and be prepared. Intravascular volume needs to be more than adequate. Before removal of the cross-clamp, have additional volume available, especially colloid. Red cells and other blood products are often necessary.

Transplant Surgery

You probably won't get to do a transplant case until you've been around the OR for a year or two, not so much because they are hard cases in sick patients (they are) but because everyone involved will want things to go perfectly. Transplant surgeons are perfectionists and will tend to be more involved in your business than the average operator. Your staff anesthesiologist will want to preserve face with the surgeon. And the patient will have spent half a lifetime in the medical system and will typically be informed and anxious.

Transplant patients are typically summoned to the hospital on a moment's notice, often straight from their lavish breakfasts. They will all have full stomachs, be extremely anxious, and be so sick medically that a rapid-sequence induction will be out of the question. Remember to give aspiration prophylaxis!

Anesthetically your goal will be to keep the patient well perfused. The surgeon will urge you to keep the patient well hydrated and will frown on the use of vasoconstrictive agents such as phenylephrine or norepinephrine. Inotropes such as dopamine are preferred, with the object of keeping the cardiac output high. Bleeding may be brisk, and you may have to start transfusing early and then work hard to keep ahead.

The new organ, whatever it is, is put in cold and will be loaded with metabolic by-products. When the vascular clamps are removed and the organ is reperfused, all of this garbage will be washed back into the circulation. Arrhythmias, systemic hypotension, and pulmonary hypertension can all result and may sometimes be severe. Having the patient warm and volume replete before the clamp comes off is your best defense.

Immunosuppressive and antibiotic drug recommendations are changing too fast for the nonspecialist to keep track. Give the patient what the surgeon says to give when he or she says to give it. Antibiotics may affect neuromuscular blockade (something you're probably already used to) and occasionally blood pressure. Immunosuppressives generally have little effect on the anesthetic, although corticosteroids will increase serum glucose. The lifelong immunosuppression confronting the patient means that you must pay strict attention to sterile technique during all of your procedures.

Organ Harvest

Description: A brain-dead body is transported from the ICU to the OR, where all the vital organs are summarily removed. The kidneys and pancreas go first, followed by the liver, the heart, and the lungs, more or less in that order. (The skin, corneas, and bone go next, but you'll be long gone by that point.)

Position:	Supine
Estimated time:	4 hours
Estimated blood loss:	Infinite
Need for muscle relaxation:	Required
Indicated monitors:	Standard, Foley, A-line; consider CVP/PA
Postoperative analgesia:	Not applicable
Acceptable techniques:	Support only

Comments: This is a complex case, frequently handed to the most junior person on the call team, since it's usually the middle of the night and the downside to the patient is minimal. The patient will not survive the procedure in any case.

You will probably receive a variety of instructions from the harvesting surgeon(s) about how they want the patient maintained. If multiple harvesters disagree about some aspect of management, make them work it out among themselves.

In general, if the blood pressure falls you should consider an inotrope (like dopamine) before a vasoconstrictor (phenylephrine or norepinephrine) to maintain perfusion of the organs being harvested.

Maintain strict sterile technique throughout. All of the organs will be going to immunosuppressed patients.

Living Related Kidney Donation

Description: The kidney is accessed through a lateral flank incision and the ureter, vein, and artery are ligated. The organ is then removed and taken into the next OR over, where it is installed in a waiting recipient.

Position:	Lateral decubitus, table flexed, kidney rest up
Estimated time:	3 hours
Estimated blood loss:	500 ml; type and cross-match 2 units
Need for muscle relaxation:	Required for exposure
Indicated monitors:	Standard, Foley, A-line
Postoperative analgesia:	IV
Acceptable techniques:	GETA, combined

Comments: These patients are usually young and healthy, but very, very nervous. Be generous with the sedation preoperatively.

Do your best for the departing kidney: keep the patient well hydrated, and keep perfusion pressure up. Avoid vasoconstricting agents such as phenylephrine.

Follow urine output closely, but don't expect a big change when the kidney is removed. If the patient can't get by pretty well on just one kidney, then someone has made a tremendous mistake.

After flattening out the bed (which helps the surgeon close the wound) you can extubate the patient on his or her side, allowing any secretions to drain harmlessly (but inaesthetically) out the mouth.

Kidney Transplant

Description: A kidney arrives packed in ice and is then implanted in the left or right iliac fossa. The renal artery and vein are grafted to the iliac vessels and then the ureter is either implanted directly into the bladder or else joined end-to-end to the native ureter (the native kidney having been removed first).

Position:	Supine, one hip bumped up
Estimated time:	5 hours
Estimated blood loss:	1,000 ml; type and cross-match 4 units
Need for muscle relaxation:	Required
Indicated monitors:	Standard, Foley, A-line; consider CVP
Postoperative analgesia:	III
Acceptable techniques:	GETA, combined

Comments: These patients are often quite debilitated, having been on dialysis for months to years. Determine when the last dialysis was and make sure you check the labs carefully. It's very unlikely the surgery will be canceled for an abnormal lab value, but at least you'll know what to worry about. The procedure will be longer and bloodier if a nephrectomy is included, although the ureteral hook-up will be easier for the surgeon.

Your hemodynamic goal should be to maintain a high perfusion pressure throughout. Keep the patient well hydrated, use inotropic rather than vasoconstrictive agents to support the pressure, and transfuse early.

On the other hand, remember that if the transplant doesn't work, the patient will have no way to get rid of all of that excess fluid. This is why many anesthetists (and transplant surgeons) will prefer to use colloid rather than crystalloid to maintain intravascular volume.

When the artery and vein are connected, there will be a "shock load" to the heart as all of the cold, ischemic factor–filled perfusate washes into the circulation. This will cause a sudden drop in pressure and occasionally a drop in pulmonary compliance. Both will be short-lived, so don't overreact.

The surgeons will typically ask for furosemide and mannitol doses shortly after the new kidney is connected. Follow their instructions, but don't be surprised if the new kidney doesn't do much for the first hour or so. It takes a while for it to warm up and start making urine.

Pancreas Transplant

Description: Through a low abdominal incision the pancreas is grafted to the iliac vessels and the pancreatic duct is connected to the bladder (so that digestive enzymes can drain harmlessly out of the body).

Position:	Supine
Estimated time:	5 hours
Estimated blood loss:	500 ml; type and cross-match 2 units
Need for muscle relaxation:	Required
Indicated monitors:	Standard, Foley, A-line
Postoperative analgesia:	III
Acceptable techniques:	GETA, combined

Comments: This operation is done in end-stage diabetics who may be in rocky shape preoperatively. Check the labs carefully, remember to consider your insulin dose, and plan on measuring glucose intraoperatively.

This operation is commonly combined with a kidney transplant from the same host. The joint operation takes about 7 hours and is more tedious than truly life-threatening. Good IV access and monitoring are required.

As with all transplants, maintenance of an adequate perfusion pressure is essential. Transfuse early and often, and work to keep the intravascular volume and urine output high.

The native pancreas is left carefully alone.

Liver Transplant

Description: The surgeon makes a huge chevron incision in the upper abdomen and dissects down to the porta hepatis. The hepatic artery, portal vein, proximal and distal inferior vena cava (IVC), and bile duct are all clamped, and the old liver is removed. The new liver is dropped in the hole, and the hepatic artery is connected along with the proximal and distal IVC and the portal vein. The liver is then reperfused while the surgeons work out the biliary anastomosis, which goes either end-to-end with the old bile duct or into a Roux-en-Y segment of jejunum.

Position:	Supine
Estimated time:	8 hours
Estimated blood loss:	5,000 ml; type and cross-match 10 units PRBCs, 10 units fresh-frozen plasma, 10 units platelets
Need for muscle relaxation:	Required
Indicated monitors:	Standard, Foley, A-line, PA, frequent blood samples
Postoperative analgesia:	IV
Acceptable techniques:	GETA, combined

Comments: This patient will be sick to start with; check the preoperative labs carefully. All patients will be somewhat coagulopathic. The most difficult are patients with portal hypertension: Everything the surgeons dissect in the belly will bleed.

This case is basically a bloodbath. Have abundant IV access available (we use three PA introducers: one in each internal jugular and one in the antecubital vein), have a heated rapid infusion device, and make sure the blood bank stays well ahead of you.

Keep the anesthetic simple. Give a big slug of narcotics up front, keep the patient paralyzed, and don't plan to extubate for several days. If you do put an epidural in at the start, don't use it until you're sure all the bleeding has stopped.

Find out whether your surgeons will need the left arm for a bypass infuser. Femoral or portal vein to left axillary vein bypass is used to decompress the liver and lower extremities during clamping of the IVC.

Reperfusing the new liver will dump a large load of toxins directly into the heart. This occasionally causes a complete arrest if the potassium load is high enough and will always cause some amount of instability. Crank the pressure way up before the surgeons open, have inotropic agents available, and expect a rocky ride.

Heart Transplant

Description: The chest is opened, bypass is established, and the old heart is removed at a line halfway across the atria. The remaining atrial flaps are sewn to the transplanted atria, the great vessels are connected, the patient is warmed, the fingers are crossed, and separation from bypass is attempted.

Position:	Supine
Estimated time:	6 hours
Estimated blood loss:	2,000 ml; type and cross-match 10 units, platelets, fresh-frozen plasma, cryoprecipitate
Need for muscle relaxation:	Required
Indicated monitors:	Standard, Foley, A-line, CVP or PA; consider TEE
Postoperative analgesia:	IV
Acceptable techniques:	High-dose narcotics/GETA

Comments: This case is often done in "off hours." Although the lines can go in, induction must await the go-ahead from the harvesting surgeon.

Although the patient may be very nervous, myocardial depressants should be carefully avoided. These patients typically have very low ejection fractions and no cardiac reserve.

Central lines should be placed from the left internal jugular, saving the right internal jugular for the multiple endocardial biopsies to come.

Weaning from bypass may be complicated by right heart failure precipitated by difficulty in adequately protecting the right heart. Treat with hyperventilation and pulmonary vasodilators (isoproterenol or prostaglandin E_1). Consider running any necessary vasoconstrictors (like norepinephrine) through a left atrial line where they will not affect the right heart. A-V node dysfunction may necessitate A-V pacing.

Plan on a lot more bleeding than in a normal valve or coronary artery bypass grafting because of the extent of exposed suture lines, the length of the bypass run, pre-operative anticoagulants, and the mild liver failure common in these patients. Be ready with your big guns as soon as the patient is off bypass.

As with most cardiac surgeries, plan to keep the patient anesthetized and ventilated for at least 24 hours postoperatively.

Lung Transplant

Description: Through a transverse thoracotomy extended to the right side, the surgeon dissects free the existing right lung and removes it. The new lung is installed, and the artery and veins are hooked up. The lung is then perfused while the bronchial anastomosis is being completed. A flap of omentum is typically brought up from the belly to wrap around the bronchial anastomosis.

Position:	Supine
Estimated time:	6 hours
Estimated blood loss:	500 ml plus; type and crossmatch 4 units; have fresh-frozen plasma and platelets ready
Need for muscle relaxation:	Required
Indicated monitors:	Standard, Foley, A-line, PA, frequent ABGs
Postoperative analgesia:	IV
Acceptable techniques:	GETA, epidural for postop use

Comments: Patients typically have alpha$_1$-antitrypsin disease, idiopathic pulmonary hypertension, or cystic fibrosis (double-lung transplants). Their exercise tolerance preoperatively will be near zero. Unperfused lung has an extremely short life span, so that one or more potential recipients are usually admitted and lined up before the tissue typing is complete, let alone the lung harvest. These patients will often come in, get lined and premedicated, and then go home when the tissue type is wrong or the potential lung turns out to be unsuitable. Needless to say, this whole process makes them incredibly nervous.

A left-sided double-lumen tube is required for both right single-lung and double-lung transplants. (The surgeon will typically be able to do the anastomosis below the end of the tube on the left.) These patients may be very hard to ventilate adequately on one lung, often requiring your continuous personal attention and tolerance of a certain amount of hypoxia and hypercarbia.

The anesthetic should be kept very simple: fentanyl and vecuronium. Extubation will be hours to days later after the first crisis point for rejection has passed. An epidural will be a great help in managing postoperative pain and facilitating extubation.

There will be a certain amount of ischemic shock transmitted to the heart when the new lung is first perfused. Because the blood vessels are connected before the bronchus, there will also be a pretty fair $\dot{V}/\dot{Q}$ mismatch (depending on the degree of hypoxic pulmonary vasoconstriction in the new lung) until you can ventilate both lungs.

Road Trips

When in the course of anesthetic practice it becomes necessary to leave the warm confines of the operating room and take your act on the road, there are a few points you might wish to remember:

1. *You're not in Kansas anymore.* When entering someone else's turf, don't take anything for granted. Find out where the closest oxygen hook-up is; find out where the suction is; find out where you can plug yourself in. (If the answer to all three is "back in the OR," maybe that's where the patient should be as well.) Taking a good look at the setup on the night before you have to do a pediatric MRI might save you a few trips back and forth the next day.

2. *Don't count on a lot of help.* You may not think the nurses and surgeons are a whole lot of assistance when you're working in the OR, but you'll change your mind when you ask someone in the ER to give you some cricoid pressure and they look at you like you've got three heads. Either bring your own help (always a good idea) or get good at explaining exactly what you want done in a way that a complete novice could follow. Call for help early if it looks like you might want it, and make sure the folks back in the OR know where you are and what you're doing.

3. *Bring what you need.* Most anesthesia departments maintain equipment for road shows, ranging from a bag full of intubation gear to a complete anesthesia machine and cart for the MRI scanner. Make sure you're fully stocked before leaving home or you might find yourself doing a lot of improvising. If it turns out that the laryngoscope on the ward's crash cart actually works, by all means use it; it'll be one less that you have to clean. But always bring your own stuff as well to make sure that you have what you want.

4. *Expect a different sort of patient preparation.* Emergencies won't look much different, but your elective cases might. Every anesthesia department out there has had to find a mechanism for making sure that CT and MRI

kids show up in the right place at the right time with the right NPO status. Find out how your department handles these patients before doing the anesthetic. Where will the patients arrive? What paperwork will they have? Will the PACU be expecting them when you're finished?

5. *Deal with the monitors you have.* They may not be the ones you're used to, but you may not have any choice. Substandard monitoring is common outside of the OR and is one of the best reasons to refuse to do an anesthetic outside the OR. Many times, though, in the patient's best interests you will have no choice but to do the case anyway.

6. *Remember that transport can be dangerous.* Don't be the first person in your department to find yourself in a jammed elevator without a laryngoscope, without oxygen, and without a prayer. Make patients stable before you move either by anesthetizing and relaxing them thoroughly or by waiting to move until they are extubated and wide awake. Take your emergency gear with you, and make sure you have the monitors you need to keep track of the patient.

Emergency Intubation

Description: Your beeper goes off and you are summoned to the ER, the ICU, or some even less likely location to exercise your special powers of airway management. If you're lucky, it's a controlled situation in the ICU (like some congestive heart failure patient who just isn't making it); if you're unlucky, it's a total disaster (you provide the example—we're sure you've seen a few).

Position:	Supine
Estimated time:	Is it in yet?
Estimated blood loss:	Minimal
Need for muscle relaxation:	Helpful
Indicated monitors:	Whatever you can get
Postoperative analgesia:	II
Acceptable techniques:	MAC, GA

Comments: Patient disease makes a big difference in your approach to the emergency intubation. In a code situation or a bad trauma, you will simply be looking to get the tube in any way you can. In other cases you may want to move more slowly. Therefore, the first question you should ask yourself is, How long do I have to do this?

Get yourself to the head of the bed while asking what the story is. If you make eye contact with someone important as you go, you're more likely to get an intelligent answer, although probably not the whole story.

While you're thinking about your plan, take the time to get the patient into a good sniffing position (unless the cervical spine is a concern) and ventilate him or her adequately by mask with 100% oxygen. Road trip intubations are often amazingly difficult for the uninitiated, and the reason is usually the lack of a good position.

Get all the equipment you need. If you read the introduction to this chapter, then you already have it all with you; otherwise you're depending on the kindness of strangers. This includes finding the suction outlet and getting it hooked to a Yankauer sucker.

Give your anesthetic. In the code situation this means nothing. In the unstable near-code it may mean a spray of local anesthesia or a slug of IV lidocaine. In the obtunded patient it may mean just a muscle relaxant.

Rarely will it mean thiopental and succinylcholine because rarely will you have trained assistance to give cricoid pressure.

Go for it. Most near-dead patients can be intubated without muscle relaxants. Most near-near-dead patients can be easily intubated by a blind nasal approach with topical anesthesia. Your fallback position in all cases, though, including the unstable neck, is to stick a laryngoscope in and follow it with an oral tube. If you can't get it after a pass or two, call for help and ask for a tracheostomy. Hypoxia kills people quickly.

Once the tube is in, your job is essentially done, although you might want to hang around and try to scoop up a central line. After verifying bilateral breath sounds, turn the tube over to the respiratory therapist for taping and hand ventilation until a mechanical ventilator is available. Write a brief note on the chart.

CT Scan

Description: The patient is placed on the gantry of the machine, taped in position, and then moved into the doughnut for the actual scan.

Position:	Usually supine
Estimated time:	45 minutes
Estimated blood loss:	Zero
Need for muscle relaxation:	None
Indicated monitors:	Standard
Postoperative analgesia:	I
Acceptable techniques:	GETA or heavy sedation

Comments: These patients may be children of any age with a wide range of congenital anomalies. (Or else why are you scanning them?) They may also be belligerent drunk motor vehicle accident victims from the ER or ICU. Your mission is to make the patient hold still for the scan in whatever way you can. A CT is less sensitive than an MRI but still requires stillness for each image.

Be wary of the patient who is "too sick to sedate": one with an intracranial mass and elevated intracranial pressure (ICP) who may become sedated all too easily. Sedation leads to respiratory depression, which leads to increased CO_2, which leads to an increase in ICP, which leads to more sedation, which leads to.... Here in the northern hemisphere these patients will have a tendency to go down the drain clockwise.

CTs can often be accomplished with heavy sedation but will sometimes require a general anesthetic. Access to the patient will be difficult because the scanner is in the way, so you'll want to make sure you're happy with the anesthetic before allowing the scan to start (and removing yourself from the radiation-filled immediate vicinity). A continuous infusion of propofol or methohexital is better than repeated IV doses.

If you are scanning an intubated patient from the ICU or ER, make sure you contact respiratory therapy beforehand to arrange for a ventilator in the CT scan room. You will probably not want to bring your anesthesia machine there for a patient who can be easily managed with IV agents. Also be careful with patient transport; use a

monitor and supplemental oxygen if the patient is still sedated postprocedure.

Some scans require the injection of iodinated contrast material, which has a propensity for causing allergic reactions. Have the appropriate emergency drugs handy.

MRI Scan

Description: The patient is anesthetized, shifted to the gantry of the MRI scanner, secured in place with all appropriate monitoring, and the scan is begun. Your credit cards are simultaneously erased. That is all.

Position:	Supine, with airway 10 feet from anesthesia provider
Estimated time:	1 hour
Estimated blood loss:	Zero
Need for muscle relaxation:	None
Indicated monitors:	Standard
Postoperative analgesia:	I
Acceptable techniques:	GETA

Comments: Your patients will range from otherwise normal but claustrophobic adults all the way down to severely anomalous infants.

Your mission is to make the patient hold still, since even the slightest movement might wash out the whole study. An MRI will frequently require a general anesthetic, partly because of the length and noise of the procedure, partly because the patient will be 6 feet up the tube of the machine from you. Make sure that all of your anesthetic equipment and monitors are MRI-compatible. Check oxygen and nitrous hook-ups and the availability of suction equipment. Do all of this *before* the patient arrives.

Typically you will induce general anesthesia, start your IV, and intubate the patient on the stretcher, then move the patient to the gantry of the scanner. Make sure you have enough slack in your tubes and wires to reach all the way into the machine. Spontaneous ventilation is something to strive for, as it gives you one more monitor of anesthetic depth and allows patients to titrate their own anesthetic depth when you are using a volatile anesthetic. Your end-tidal CO_2 monitor will be sipping through a 20-foot hose, so it won't be quantitatively accurate. However, a wave form does indicate continued ventilation.

Anything metallic is a big problem for the MRI scanner. Loose metal, like laryngoscope blades, scissors, or stethoscopes, will fly toward the magnet, damaging it or anything that gets in the way. Metal attached to the patient—ECG leads, hip pins, surgical staples—may heat up and cause an injury.

Not only will your credit cards erase (and your pocket calculator, and your watch, and your beeper), but your monitors may also have trouble with the magnetic fields. Oximeters must be specially constructed to work with the MRI, and capnometer and blood pressure cables will have to extend out of the room to their base units (make sure you can see the numbers from wherever you end up standing). An ECG may be completely impossible, and you may just have to do without.

There's nothing harmful about staying in the scan room with the patient (as far as we know now), although it can be pretty loud. You're closer if anything happens, and you can keep a better eye on the patient's ventilation. Just make sure you can see all the monitors you have, and ask the technician to let you know when the end of the scan is approaching.

Gadolinium is given as an IV contrast agent for some studies. As far as we can tell, it has no effect on your anesthetic.

Know how to get at the patient's airway in a hurry. There's normally a manual override lever that lets you pull the patient out of the scanner, if you have to. Know where this is and how it works.

Transport from the MRI to the PACU can be an exciting adventure. Provide supplemental oxygen, use a transport monitor if the patient is not wide awake, and carry emergency drugs and airway equipment with you.

Upper Endoscopy

Description: The surgeons stick a very large fiberoptic scope down the patient's throat and examine the esophagus, the stomach, and the first part of the duodenum. Biopsies and cautery are also possible through the scope.

Position:	Lateral "park bench"
Estimated time:	60 minutes
Estimated blood loss:	Zero
Need for muscle relaxation:	None
Indicated monitors:	Standard
Postoperative analgesia:	I; nothing
Acceptable techniques:	Usually local plus IV sedation

Comments: Only the sicker patients will tend to come to your attention, since the majority of these procedures are done in the clinic or outpatient center without your involvement. The patient you get to monitor will be bleeding heavily from his esophageal varices, an ASA IV from his heart condition, afflicted with senile dementia, or all three.

Pay attention to the surgeon as he topicalizes the upper airway. You might learn something.

Beware of oversedating. Once the topicalization hits, there really isn't much stimulation provided by the procedure. Make sure that you are providing supplemental oxygen, and take your monitoring seriously. The less anesthesia you give, the better.

Examining the lower esophagus can irritate the next organ forward, which is the heart. Beware of sudden arrhythmias.

Dreaded complications of perforating the stomach or esophagus include pneumothorax, infection, severe bleeding, and—usually—emergency surgery. Pay close attention to what your surgeon is biopsying.

Cardioversion

Description: You are dispatched to the cardiac care unit to anesthetize a patient for the millisecond it takes to defibrillate from supraventricular tachycardia or atrial fibrillation back to sinus rhythm. Unfortunately, that millisecond is fairly stimulating.

Position:	Supine
Estimated time:	10 minutes
Estimated blood loss:	None
Need for muscle relaxation:	None
Indicated monitors:	ECG, oximeter, blood pressure
Postoperative analgesia:	I
Acceptable techniques:	GA, MAC

Comments: The typical patient will be a 65-year-old man with new-onset atrial fibrillation that has been rate-controlled by digoxin but not converted. There are obviously lots of other indications for electrical defibrillation, but in most of those cases the patient will be unstable and the cardiologists won't wait to call you before zapping. (As a corollary, if you ever arrive to find the patient unstable, don't aggravate things by adding an anesthetic agent. Just tell them to fire away—and then go home and tell your aging relatives not to get sick in that neighborhood.)

Ideally the patient is NPO. If not, you will generally weigh the risks and benefits and decide that you still don't want to intubate but will just make your sedation a little lighter.

Preoxygenate with your bag and mask.

We generally use just enough propofol (if otherwise healthy) or etomidate (if not) to get the patient's eyes closed, then tell the cardiologist to fire away. Some groaning and patient movement will still occur with the defibrillation, but vital signs will remain stable and the patient will have no recall. Usually the first two attempts at cardioversion will fit into the initial dose of amnestic; if further attempts are needed, you may need to redose.

Between shocks you should support the patient's airway and ventilate him or her gently with the bag and mask if needed. Most of the time patients will be breathing on their own without a whole lot of help. Once they can also support their own airway you can put a face mask on them and get yourself out of there.

Don't touch the bed or the patient when they're zapping (you probably already knew that). If ventricular tachycardia or ventricular fibrillation occur, support the airway and proceed with advanced cardiac life support.

Pacemaker Insertion

Description: The pacemaker leads are threaded percutaneously into the heart from the subclavian artery and positioned under fluoroscopy. The generator box is inserted into a small subcutaneous pocket on the chest wall and programmed and tested via a computer control box and magnet.

Position:	Supine
Estimated time:	60 minutes
Estimated blood loss:	Minimal
Need for muscle relaxation:	None
Indicated monitors:	Standard
Postoperative analgesia:	II
Acceptable techniques:	MAC, GETA

Comments: You'll only see the really sick patients for this procedure since most of the time the cardiologists will do it themselves under local anesthesia.

The sick ones are actually easy to manage: Don't give them anything that might potentially be a negative inotrope or a sedative. Let the surgeon give the local while you concentrate on the hand-holding. There's no anesthesia like no anesthesia!

All kinds of rhythms can pop up while the cardiologist is attempting to get the leads positioned correctly. Ask for a halt if things get really ugly; usually the heart will settle down when you're not messing with it. Otherwise follow the cardiologist's advice regarding antiarrhythmics and defibrillation. Your job is to tell him when things are bad. His job is to fix it.

And while you're at it, why not ask the cardiologist what kind of pacemaker is being implanted, how it will be programmed, and what effect a magnet will have on it. Then write this information in the patient's chart, where the next anesthesia resident can find it easily.

Closed Reduction of Fracture/ Relocation of Dislocated Joint

Description: The surgeon straightens out the problem, using x-ray or fluoroscopy to verify that everything is back where it belongs.

Position:	As needed (most often supine)
Estimated time:	15 minutes
Estimated blood loss:	Zero
Need for muscle relaxation:	Helpful
Indicated monitors:	Standard
Postoperative analgesia:	II
Acceptable techniques:	GA, regional, MAC

Comments: Sometimes this procedure can be done under heavy sedation, using a benzodiazepine to confer some amount of muscle relaxation. This is what the surgeon is hoping when he asks you to come down to the ER to give him a hand. This obviously works best with very short procedures such as relocating a dislocated hip, knee, or shoulder.

This tends to be an emergency procedure so that full stomach considerations apply. Very heavy sedation or general anesthesia probably mandates an endotracheal tube.

Closed fracture reductions in particular may become open procedures. Percutaneous pinning to secure the fracture counts as an open procedure and necessitates a serious regional or general anesthetic.

Frequent x-rays are common.

Don't forget to check the patient's secondary trauma assessment. Did he also hit his head when he fell? Avoid embarrassment and think carefully about the mechanism of injury before starting your anesthetic.

Lithotripsy

Description: An ultrasonic wave generator is focused through the skin on a kidney stone (under fluoroscopic guidance) and is fired several hundred times. The stone breaks into small pieces and is flushed out of the renal pelvis.

Position:	Supine or semi-Fowler's
Estimated time:	1 hour
Estimated blood loss:	None
Need for muscle relaxation:	None
Indicated monitors:	Standard; waterproof ECG leads required with older lithotripsy machines
Postoperative analgesia:	II; renal colic pain, PO medications
Acceptable techniques:	Epidural, spinal, GETA, or MAC

Comments: Older lithotripsy machines require the patient to be immersed in a large steel bathtub, raising an interesting set of issues for the anesthetist:

1. The patient has to be anesthetized and then moved into this position.
2. Immersion can cause vasodilatation and vagal responses.
3. Monitoring can be difficult. Waterproof tape is needed over the ECG pads. The arms are usually supported outside the tub. Watch for brachial plexus injuries.
4. Real anesthesia is needed with this technology (not MAC).

Newer lithotripsy machines allow the patient to lie supine on a water mattress and allow MACs or straight local procedures.

With either technique it is important to keep your equipment out of the path of the sound waves. The sound wave pulses are triggered by the ECG, so avoid slowing the heart rate too much or the procedure will take longer.

Frequent fluoroscopy is common.

It is not unusual to do a cystoscopy and stent place-ment prior to the lithotripsy, which may change the patient's anesthetic requirements.

Lithotripsy is typically done on an outpatient basis in otherwise healthy patients. Everyone will be expecting a simple anesthetic, so the finger-pointing will be severe if a complication occurs.

Percutaneous Nephrostomy (PCN) Tube Placement

Description: A collection of pus in the renal pelvis is aspirated percutaneously, under ultrasound guidance, and a drainage tube is then placed through the same tract.

Position:	Prone
Estimated time:	1 hour
Estimated blood loss:	Minimal
Need for muscle relaxation:	None
Indicated monitors:	Standard
Postoperative analgesia:	II; PO medications
Acceptable techniques:	Epidural, spinal, MAC, or GETA

Comments: Because of the awkward position, regional anesthesia is usually easier and quicker than a general.

This procedure can be done with just local anesthesia, but it is usually fairly painful.

Fluoroscopy with contrast material may be part of the procedure. Watch for anaphylaxis and have your epinephrine ready.

This procedure often precedes, by a day or two, a more definitive procedure to address the infected, obstructed kidney. Epidurals and monitoring lines placed for the tube placement may be left in place for the bigger operation to follow.

Electroconvulsive Therapy (ECT)

Description: Psychiatrists do this procedure to treat severe depression. An electrical current is administered to one lobe of the brain via a machine much like a defibrillator. The success of the procedure can depend on the length and intensity of the seizure that follows the shock.

Position:	Supine
Estimated time:	15 minutes
Estimated blood loss:	Zero
Need for muscle relaxation:	Required
Indicated monitors:	Standard
Postoperative analgesia:	I
Acceptable techniques:	GA

Comments: Typically the patient receives a short general anesthetic by mask, with propofol, thiopental, etomidate, or methohexital. Emergency airway equipment should be close at hand, however, and you should check your oxygen supply and suction before you start.

Aspiration prophylaxis is recommended.

A special bite-block designed to protect the patient's teeth may also be used, just in case the succinylcholine doesn't prevent all of the seizing.

Applying direct current to the brain produces a variety of short-lived but exciting hemodynamic effects. Bradycardia is common, sometimes followed by tachycardia and severe dysrhythmias. Transient hypertension is common. These are best treated with esmolol but only after the initial bradycardia has gone by (yes, we learned this the hard way). Have atropine available just in case.

Typically a given patient will have a series of ECTs over weeks to months. Tachyphylaxis to the shock may develop, manifested by diminishing returns to the electrical stimulation. Caffeine may be administered to enhance seizure activity (it also enhances tachyarrhythmias), and we have found that changing anesthetic agents may also help. This is an issue to talk over with the psychiatrists before you start.

Muscle relaxation (typically with succinylcholine) is required to keep patients from hurting themselves when they seize. Typically a tourniquet is inflated on one extremity just prior to the succinylcholine so that the shrinks can judge the seizure activity by watching that limb twitch while the rest of the patient remains flaccid.

Neuroembolization

Description: In the angiography suite the neuroradiologist identifies the blood supply to a tumor, arteriovenous malformation (AVM), or aneurysm, gets as close to it as possible with a catheter, and then injects it with some instantly coagulating compound. Sometimes this achieves a complete cure (as with AVMs). Other times it works to reduce bleeding at a subsequent definitive surgery. Sometimes it doesn't work at all. It always takes a long time.

Position:	Supine
Estimated time:	2 hours plus
Estimated blood loss:	Minimal
Need for muscle relaxation:	None
Indicated monitors:	Standard
Postoperative analgesia:	I
Acceptable techniques:	MAC, GETA

Comments: MAC is desirable because, on the one hand, the radiologist likes to have the patient awake enough to tell him if he suddenly strokes (it happens), and on the other hand, likes to have the patient comfortable enough to tolerate the injections—which can cause a very painful burning sensation—without a lot of moving around. Your presence is especially constructive if the lesion being embolized is in a sensitive area, and hemodynamic perturbations are anticipated.

General anesthesia may be necessary from the outset if the radiologist needs you to control the patient's ventilation so he can see what he's doing. That is common with lesions of the thoracic spine. More often, though, general anesthesia becomes a requirement after several hours of gradually deepening sedation. Make sure before starting that you have all of the drugs and equipment (including your anesthesia machine) you will need when this happens.

Talk to the radiologist or the technicians to figure out how you can get to the patient's head in an emergency. If nothing else, it will let them know that an emergency is possible and that they'd better believe you if you say that you need to get to the patient.

Hemodynamic stimulation is impressive with intra-arterial injections but usually very short-lived. In potentially unstable patients you may want an arterial line and some vasoactive substances on hand to manage these procedures. Esmolol, phenylephrine, and nitroprusside are all quite useful.

These cases can arise as emergencies. If you find yourself doing general anesthesia on some sick patient in the middle of the night four floors from your OR, make sure you know where your backup is and how long it'll take him or her to get to you.

Pediatric Cardiac Catheterization

Description: The arterial and venous systems are cannulated from the groin, and contrast injections are used to define the exact anatomy of the heart and central vessels. General anesthesia or heavy sedation is required to keep the child still during the procedure.

Position:	Supine
Estimated time:	60 minutes
Estimated blood loss:	Minimal
Need for muscle relaxation:	Helpful
Indicated monitors:	Standard
Postoperative analgesia:	II
Acceptable techniques:	GETA

Comments: We really don't want to get into all of the possible congenital cardiac anomalies here; whole textbooks have been written on the subject. Suffice it to say that your patient will have one of them (or maybe several) and you should be aware of how to manage it.

At a guess, your best policy is to keep the patient as close as possible to his or her baseline values. This can be difficult while trying to get an uncooperative child sedated and intubated, but if it were easy they wouldn't need someone so talented to do it.

In general, congenital anomalies break down into those that cause a right-to-left shunt, and therefore desaturation, and those that cause a left-to-right shunt, and therefore pulmonary overload. The latter category, which includes patent ductus arteriosus and small atrioseptal defects and ventroseptal defects, will probably bother you less. Most of these patients will not become clinically ill until much later in life, when pulmonary hypertension begins to develop.

The fun for you will come in the cyanotic group. If a patient begins to desaturate on you, you should keep two cardinal principles in mind: lower the pulmonary resistance and raise the systemic. A Valsalva maneuver works for Fallot's tetralogy kids, and you can do the same thing with a little phenylephrine. Oxygen and hyperventilation are good too.

Remember that the little tykes might have associated congenital anomalies and really scary airways. Get help early if desaturation or bradycardia occur.

Wear lead when the cardiologist is fluoroscoping.

See also the section on pediatric cardiac catheterization in Chapter 15.

Index